# *21 Sleeps*

## *Lessons of a Lifetime*

*Aislinn Cambridge*

*Dedicated to the amazing, inspiring people who have touched my life.*

*Especially to the memory of the late Johnny Twohig (The Squire)*

*Love and gratitude to all my teachers and students in the school of life*

*Chapter 1 - Sleep One*

*Thursday, October 24th*

It was the worst time that I can remember. The weather was what we call 'real Irish' – It was cold, wet and windy and seemed to match my mood perfectly.

I rolled over in bed, turning my back on the world, and lay there listening to the sound of the rain against the window. I just wanted to go to sleep. Considering I hadn't slept in days, that was probably understandable.

But on this particular day, like it or not, I had to get up and face the world. It was October 24th...exactly two days after my best friend Jake had died.

Jake wasn't much older than me and we'd been best friends since we were kids. We had done everything together; learning to walk, to cycle a bike, to climb a tree, to run away from home. You name it, we had done it. When he died, I was a mess.

Somehow, eventually, I managed to drag myself out of the bed. I remember very clearly that I started to hum *Galileo*, one of Jake's favourite songs. It was lodged in my head and the only way to get it out was to let it out. I hummed and hummed, and began to think of what we would have been doing differently that day if he were alive.

5

I glanced at my phone several times, remembering the messages he used to send me most mornings. They were always full of positivity and encouragement. 'Have a super day Shell and remember we don't get older, we get better :-)' I needed one of those messages now more than ever.

I made my way towards the wardrobe to look for something to wear, which triggered memories of how Jake would have given a little speech about being organised, especially the night before a major event. He would say that it would eliminate unnecessary stress in the morning and boy, was he right. It was typical of him; he was always organised and well prepared. In fact, he was on to something there because I never really saw him stressed out. I managed to pull myself together, and just as I was making my way downstairs the phone rang. I won't lie; I got a little fright. I think in a silly way I half-believed it was Jake.

"Hello"

"Hey Shell, I was just calling to see if you needed a lift to the church?"

It was Robert, my ex-boyfriend and a mutual friend of Jake's.

"No thanks Rob, Eve is picking me up."

"Right. Of course. So… how are you holding up?"

"Look, Rob, thanks for the call, but Eve's outside so I'll have to go. I will see you at the funeral, okay?"

He started to respond, but I hung up. I placed the phone on the work top, then slid down the side of the kitchen press and started to cry for the first time since I had heard that Jake was dead. Samantha, Jake's sister, was the one who called me that evening to tell me he had been in a crash. He was actually on his way to my house when it happened.

It had been yet another wet evening and he had phoned me to say he was running late. He'd been playing football and, because of the torrential rain, he was giving a few of the lads a lift home on his way. He had dropped them all home and was taking the back roads to my house when a van took a corner too wide, head-on into his car. Jake died on impact.

The accident happened only five minutes from my home. As I lay up against the kitchen press crying, my sister arrived and made her way towards the sound of my sobbing.

She looked down at me and smiled. It was one of those looks that said: "I'm half sad for you and I'm half sorry for you." She sat down on the floor next to me and put her arms around me.

"I know it hurts right now," she whispered, "and you miss him, but it won't always be this hard. I promise. I think if Jake were here he'd give you one of his speeches. 'We're all going to die and that's sad, but the saddest thing is some of us never live.'" I had to laugh, mainly at Eve's really bad impersonation.

"I know! I know! It just hurts so much. I mean, it's his birthday today. Oh my God, Eve! He is being buried on his birthday!"

I could see Eve's eyes filling up and I know as much as she was trying to mind me, she wasn't strong enough to mind us both. Nobody could, in that kind of situation.

7

"I know. But knowing Jake, he would want us to celebrate his life...don't you think? Besides, we have to pull it together for a little bit; especially you! You have the eulogy to do and I know it's important to you to do it. Today, everyone needs to hear how amazing he was, and no one can tell that as well as you. Let's go and make him proud, okay?"

We got up from the floor. I grabbed my bag and an umbrella and we made our way to the car.

Traffic was much busier than usual as we drove to the local church. It didn't take us long to figure out that it was Jake's fault. It was as if the whole county was at his funeral, and not just the whole town. The church car park was completely full, so Eve suggested parking in the nearby graveyard and walking to the church.

We put up the umbrella and made our way towards the front of the church, where our family was standing. My Dad hugged me as my mother struggled to speak through her tears. My family, the Morrisseys, and Jake's family, the Lawlor's, had always been very close. I can't remember a time when they weren't around. Our families were an extension of each other and everyone in Castletown knew it. The community was close-knit. We all knew each other. There wasn't a person living there who didn't know Jake. He was the guy who was always in good humour, who always made an effort. He always left a good impression.

Jake had always been active on the local sports scene. He played everything; football, rugby, golf, boxing...before he passed, his job had been writing for a local newspaper, where he had a sports column.

8

The Lawlor family were known for their good looks and Jake was no exception. The girls in school tormented me about him when we were growing up. He was tall, dark and handsome, but to me, he was always just Jake.

He had been a rock. My safe haven. He was there for me when I'd ended it with Rob earlier that year. Looking back, I saw how he had been so good to me even though he had split from his girlfriend of two years only a few months before. He was always the brave one. He always stuck to his guns and finished what he started. I, on the other hand, finished nothing. Jake loved to point out that my creative side always got the better of my logical side. He would say that was the reason I lacked structure and organisation. He would joke about it, saying it was the reason why we were such good friends: we were polar opposites. We were yin and yang.

At the church, Father Murphy walked solemnly to the altar, the congregation standing as he entered. As he approached the pulpit, he looked around at the crowd that had turned up to pay their respects.

"Today we mourn a tragic loss," he began. "But we also celebrate a tremendous life, because Jake Lawlor was full of life."

I couldn't avoid drifting off into a daze. *Galileo* passed through my head and I thought "why do I keep hearing that song?" My introspection overpowered the moment and I didn't even realise I was being called up to speak until my Mum nudged me.

"Shell, are you okay to do this?"

"Yeah. Of course."

I stood up, still dazed, and walked to the top of the church, towards the lectern. I looked at Father Murphy as he gave me a warm, encouraging smile. I turned to the congregation and took a breath. I remember looking out and seeing so many faces, some family, some friends, work colleges, strangers, but we were all there for one reason. I took another deep breath.

"I must admit that when I sat down to write this, I couldn't help thinking about how this would have been one of the things that Jake would be far better at than me," I told them. "That's just one of the many things that separate Jake from anybody I have ever known. He was ridiculously good at everything. I know that most of you here today who knew Jake completely understand what I am saying. If I am honest, I found it quite difficult at times, I even got annoyed by it, occasionally! I remember times when Jake would become so involved in something that I became concerned for him. But he always came out on top having accomplished his goal, whether it was boxing, piano, learning Spanish, archery... chess! Anything. Everything.

"I recall once how he learned a song on the guitar in one month. That was his goal; learn a song on the guitar. He'd never played the guitar before. Now, those of you who knew Jake well know he could sing, but when I say he learned a song on guitar, I mean the boy *knew* it and played it so well you'd swear he had written it himself! That's just the way he was. His passion and drive were infectious and he inspired everyone around him. Actually, now that I think of it, I don't think he ever bothered to learn another song on guitar after that one. He said he only needed one party piece.

"I think it's also safe to say that his nickname, which he gave himself, by the way, was very well suited to him. Super! He said it so much he believed it. It was like a mantra to him, rather than a response to a question. I remember Mary telling me one time, that he'd told her that if someone asked him how he was and he answered anything besides 'Super', he felt all wrong. Isn't that right Mary?"

I looked down at Jake's mum in the front row and all of a sudden I was pulled back to the church as if I had been somewhere else the whole time I was talking. I started to feel light-headed and overwhelmed, but I carried on because I had more things to say before I was done.

"I know that Jake's family, especially his mum Mary, his sister Sam and his brother Michael, have lost a wonderful son and brother. I know I already miss his face, his voice and the warm feeling he carried with him. I believe all of us feel the same loss today. I have known Jake for as long as I can remember. Even as kids, he always had a caring and generous nature. I think what stands out more than anything about him is that he always believed that there was something special about every person. As we grew up, Jake never let go of this belief. I watched my best friend become everyone's best friend. If Jake met someone, even once, they'd call him their friend.

"He just had a way with people. He looked, he listened and he embraced each person. He would joke that he wanted to be a people

11

millionaire. I can see clearly today that, in his too short a life, he had already accomplished that. He was a go-getter. He would say 'all you have to do is decide what you want and with the inspired action, it will come.' He made it sound so simple. He made it look simple, too. Everything he wanted, he eventually accomplished. He never gave up or lost faith in himself. He used to say 'I don't want a load of I shoulda's at the end of my days.' I shoulda done this or I shoulda done that.

"Jake just grabbed life by the horns and went for it, regardless of the consequences. He was fun and energetic to be around, and he was wise and inspirational.

"That's why we will all miss him: because he lived life to the fullest and everyone around him felt it. Jake Lawlor was a friend to all. He was generous, kind, caring and open-minded. He used to say, 'it's fine being sceptical, but don't be narrow-minded.' He said and did so many wonderful things in such a short life. I can only imagine what he could have done had he been given more time.

"We love you and miss you Jake and today we celebrate the super job you made of living. I want to finish by quoting one of Jake's favourite songs:

*When you are down and troubled,*
*And you need some loving care,*
*And nothing, nothing is going right.*
*Close your eyes and think of me and soon I will be there*
*To brighten up even your darkest nights.*
*You just call out my name, and you know wherever I am*

12

*I'll come running, to see you again.*

*Winter, Spring, Summer or Fall,*

*All you have to do is call and I'll be there,*

*Yeah, you've got a friend."*

I can still hear the sobbing, loud and echoing as I stepped down from that altar. I don't know how I managed to stay composed. I can't remember going back to my seat for the rest of the sermon. It was a complete blur.

After the mass was over, the congregation walked with heads bowed to the nearby graveyard. The coffin was shouldered by Jake's older brother Michael, his uncle Jacob, my dad Gary and Jake's friends Robert, Martin and Brian. That was the part I had dreaded most. Once that coffin goes into the ground, it's over and you will never see that person again. It feels final.

I didn't want to watch. I looked over at Jake's family; his sister Sam and his mother Mary were holding hands as tears rolled down their cheeks. I felt the grief coming from their broken hearts, more and more with every sob. Suddenly weak at the knees, I grabbed my father's arm. I couldn't bear it. I remember thinking that all I wanted to do was go to sleep and block it out. The rest of the crowd shuffled towards Jake's family to pay their condolences, as my family and I made our way out of the graveyard through the rain.

In the tradition of an Irish funeral, the next stop was the local pub, Gallagher's, which was owned by Jake's uncle, Jacob. I think every person in Castletown was there. The night was full of stories: stories about Jake as a child, Jake as a teenager and Jake as a man. Every story told was happy and fun, just like Jake. It wasn't long before the singing started and the noble call was in progress, each singer demanding a song of the next.

Jake loved the noble call, and we'd spent many years of our lives taking part in this tradition. The Lawlors are a musical bunch, and it wasn't long before Jake's brother Michael was called on to sing. A few people started shouting, "Go on Mike! Sing *Galileo*. Jake loved that one!" As Michael started to sing, I remember feeling weak. I really didn't want to make a scene, so I quietly asked Dad would he take me home. Lucky for me, Dad doesn't drink so he was always like a taxi for us. That night was no exception. "I'll drop you home, love. Come on, let's go now so we can sneak out."

On the way home in the car, Dad did most of the talking. My Dad's a very chatty man. He had been like a father to the Lawlor kids since their father died, and he'd been very close to Jake. He was feeling pain as much as the rest of us, but he put on a brave face and behaved like a strong man, the way he always did. He knew very well that I was taking it hard but he also knew I don't like to deal with stuff the same way other people do. I'm known for just brushing things under the carpet.

Since I was a child the only way to get me to be dramatic or expressive in any way was through music. I lit up when I sang. When we finally arrived at my house, Dad walked me inside. "I'm grand now Dad. I'm just so tired and all I want to do is sleep. Thanks for bringing me

14

home. Go back to the pub to Mum and the girls and I will see you tomorrow."

"Okay pet," he said, and he put his arms around me and squeezed before telling me he loved me and to get some rest.

I remember closing the door, turning off the lights and going straight upstairs to bed. My head hit the pillow and I was asleep, but just minutes later I was wide awake again and feeling surprisingly fresh as if I had slept for hours. *Galileo* was in my head again, and as I stretched out on my bed I noticed it was still dark outside. I think I turned to glance at the clock, and then I heard a familiar voice.

"Well, Miss Morrissey...are you going to get up and start living or are you going to take to the bed?"

I jumped. There in the corner, sitting in the armchair, was my dear friend Jake. As you can imagine, I was pretty shocked. Before I could get words out of my mouth, he spoke again.

"Shell, I know this is a surprise, considering I am supposed to be dead and all that. But before you say anything, let me explain."

I nodded, I think. Slowly. It's not often the dead speak. I paid close attention.

"Firstly Shell, I *am* dead, so don't get too excited. Also, when I say dead I mean what most people consider dead. But you see, the thing is we don't really die...we just kind of transcend. Do you know what I mean?"

I stared at him in complete disbelief.

"I don't know what you mean. I think I'm going crazy."

15

I started to slap myself in the face in an attempt to wake myself up.

"Stop that! You'll wake up, and I only have limited time with you!"

"What?!" I stammered. "What do you mean?"

"Well, Shell, I'm dead." He paused. "Well...kind of dead. I can only talk to you when you're asleep. If you wake yourself up you will have used up one of your sleeps."

"Oh right," I said. "I'm not going crazy at all. My dead friend is coming to talk to me, but only when I'm asleep. Right then, I get it now. That sounds so much more normal, thanks."

"Good God, Shelly, drop the attitude and listen!" the spectre in my armchair said. "I know my passing is probably hard for you to handle. Especially considering how well you handle problems anyway, not!

"I'm giving you a golden opportunity here. I want to help you sort out your life and really start to live. We've been friends a long time and to be honest while I was alive you never really listened to me, but maybe now you will. I was always picking up after your messes. I was always your person to moan to. I listened to you complain way too much and watched while you did nothing to fix your situation. And all you had to do was just look at the way I lived and do what I was doing and you would have been happy. Simple!"

I was lost for words.

"Jesus, Jake! Thanks for that. I didn't realise I was such a burden to you. Wow, I think I preferred you when you were alive. Dead Jake sucks."

16

He sighed.

"Shelly, don't make me go all soppy. You know I love you and care about you. That's why I'm here to help you! This is a second chance for you to listen to me and really hear what I'm saying. To be honest, you're not doing the best job with your life at present and I'm only being so harsh because I really want you to be happy. I think this approach is better because I tip-toed around you far too much when I was alive. And bear in mind that I understand now, better than ever, how precious our lives are, and more importantly why we live at all. So do you want my help or not? I mean I can totally go and help someone else if you feel like this won't do any good."

"Okay! Okay, Mr Sarcastic. Wow!" I adjusted myself in the bed and looked at him. "This is just weird. I mean it is so good to see you, especially after today. I thought I would never see you again but I can't help feel like it's a dream or else I'm going crazy."

"It *is* a dream, and I will come to you every time you sleep for twenty-one sleeps. Every time you fall asleep. If you take a mid-day nap, that's a sleep too. You follow me, Shell?"

"I think I get it. So it's twenty-one sleeps? God, this is so weird."

The whole thing was bizarre. I was so confused. Jake could see how I felt and he tried to relax me as much as possible.

"Shelly I don't know how else to explain this, or to make it easier to understand. Maybe I should have thought it through a little more before I appeared to you. I probably should have considered how hard this would be to accept. I suppose I was just eager to get down to business. You know me, Shell; Mr Boom-Boom! Mr Do It Now!"

"Jake," I answered; "I don't know what to think. You know me well enough to realise how sceptical I am at the best of times. It's easier for me to believe that I'm going mad or I'm sleep deprived than to believe my dead best friend is appearing to me when I fall asleep. I see dead people? I mean, really?"

"I understand that," he admitted, "but here's the thing: nobody needs to know this is happening. Only you. I strongly recommend you do not tell anyone because chances are they will think you're crazy. It's a delicate time to have this discussion with any of our families or friends, and I can guarantee they will have you certified if you do. Besides, that's why I am here now; to help you get through this time and to assist and inspire you to live a wonderful life. The kind of life everyone deserves. OK?"

All I could do was smile and nod.

"Shell, do you remember my friend Jessica Chambers from college?"

It didn't ring any bells.

"Oh, come on Shell, you remember Jess! She ended up writing a motivational book about her life, '*I'm Super, Thanks for Asking.*' She was at my 30th birthday party and she brought her friend the famous singer you like."

"Tiffany-J, now I remember her."

He smiled.

"I always remember a story she told me. It's actually in her book. It was about when her father was sick. He had bowel cancer and was undergoing treatment...he was only in his forties at the time. The treatment made him very sick and he spent a lot of his time in bed. Her mum was caring for him at home, and all the while she was still working full-time and being a mum to Jess and her sisters. One morning her mum was getting up for work. It was 6.30am and as she got out of bed and started to get ready she said 'God, I would do anything to stay in bed.' Her husband looked up at her and responded, 'I'd do anything to get out of it.'

"Jessica said that from then on, her mother looked at things a little differently. But Jess...she looked at things with a whole new perspective. She says that simple exchange changed her whole life. It was like the flip of a switch. She always said it brought her from average to super, and every day she lives that lesson. Every day she gets out of bed full of gratitude for the gift of life. Let me tell you this Shell, there are very few who live like that, yet everyone and anyone can. I lived my life with that attitude for the past ten years, and you know better than anyone what we went through with my father, but did I play the 'poor me card'? No! I choose to live my life every day as if it were my last. And it's a good job I did!"

Jake always laughed at his own humour, but I couldn't laugh at that joke and my eyes started to fill up. He stopped laughing, looked at me and smiled.

19

"Shelly, I have seen you in lots of states over the years, but very seldom have I seen you crying. It's strange to see, but maybe it's necessary."

"What do you mean?" I asked.

"Don't stop yourself, Shell! Let it out, you will feel better after you do. Everyone needs a release, but I can't go into that right now. Our time together is coming to an end for today."

"What?! But why? I don't want to wake yet!"

"Well, it's not really your choice. There are rules to this arrangement. It's nearly eight hours now that you have been asleep."

"But it feels so short, Jake. It's not enough."

"I know, but I promise that you will wake up feeling really good and every time we meet in your sleep you will wake feeling great. So I have to go but remember: we all spend most of our lives doing things because we think they will bring us happiness and that's where we have gotten it backwards. I know, I've said this to you before but this time hear me: The difference between making changes and not making them is action. Take action."

Then there was nothing but a beam of light pouring in my bedroom window, blinding me. I was still in bed, but it was morning and Jake was gone. I had to stop myself from calling his name.

"Okay, I may actually be going crazy," I said to myself. "That's the most logical explanation."

I started to think about the whole experience and I was quite surprised I remembered it so clearly, even if it had been a dream. I continued talking to myself for a while.

"I never remember dreams this clearly. He did say I would feel good, and I do, but that's probably because I got a good night's sleep for the first time in days."

I put the kettle on, walked across the kitchen and hit the button on the radio, still deep in conversation with myself about my dream experience.

"It can't have been real. I was sleep deprived, that's all!"

In the background, a familiar tremolo and pizzicato swelled from the speaker, and a warm voice began to sing.

*"Galileo fell in love as a Galilean boy..."*

I rolled my eyes, looked up at my ceiling, and sighed.

"Okay, Jake. I get it."

21

*Chapter 2 - Sleep Two*

*Friday, October 25th*


After breakfast, I decided to take Jake's advice. After all, he did say the worst that could happen is I would feel better, and I suppose that's never a bad idea.

At this point, I think I should give you a little background as to my own situation. I love music and I've always wanted to be a songwriter, but I never pursued a career in music, apart from playing in a wedding band on the weekends. I don't think that really counts. To pay my mortgage and bills, I'm an administrator at the local hospital.

I don't mind the job, but the people can be quite challenging and negative. I can still hear Jake saying "you need to get on with them or get out of there." After our discussion the night before, I think I was starting to see just how right he was. I'd taken a few days off because of his passing, and I decided this was the perfect way to start putting his theory into practice

"Yes. Today I will take action," I said as I checked myself out in the mirror before leaving the house. I drove into the city, about fifteen minutes away, and as I pulled into the car park at the shopping centre, who did I spot only my ex-boyfriend, Rob. To be honest, I had been avoiding him since the break-up, and even at the funeral, I made a point of not bumping into him.

However, today, I had a different view of things. Today, I was going to change my attitude. Besides, he was also Jake's friend and I hadn't even considered how he might have been coping. Rob and Jake were childhood buddies. Their relationship was based around sport. Rob was a rugby player and Jake and he played on the local Castletown team. Rob also happened to own the local gym.

The gym was where we first felt a spark. Jake dragged me there for a fitness kick-start – one of his many attempts to help me improve my lifestyle. After a few sessions, it was obvious that Rob and I were interested in each other, and it wasn't long before we started dating. We'd been together for two years before I decided things weren't as good as they used to be and ended it flat out, with no effort to fix things.

Jake used to say it was fear. He said I wasn't afraid of being happy but afraid of being happy and then losing it. "That's life," he said: "you've got to experience the contrast of not being happy to appreciate being happy." I could see his point, but I avoid talking about or dealing with things anyway and I let them live in my head instead. The break-up had left everyone very confused. I know Rob loved me and would have done anything for me, but at the time it didn't matter. When I made up my mind, I made up my mind. Case closed.

I got out of the car and I could see Rob walking towards the exit of the car park, so I shouted after him to hold up. He turned around, looking quite surprised.

"Hey Shell, how are you?"

"Super, Rob. You?"

23

"Really? Super?" I could tell by his tone he was shocked by my response.

"Yes! So...how are you keeping?"

"Well to be quite honest, Shell, I'm only average considering the events of the past few days, and now to top it off I'm a bit confused."

"Why are you confused?" I asked.

"All of a sudden you are speaking to me now?" was the response.

"Look, Rob, I understand. It's been hard for everyone and I know we will all miss Jake, but you know as well as I do that he wouldn't want us moping around feeling sorry for ourselves. Right?"

"Well, yes. That's true I suppose! But I was talking about...well, Shell, I'm surprised you're being so friendly and normal, despite the fact that since we split you have outright refused to talk to me. You've gone out of your way to avoid me completely for the past two months."

He stared at me, looking for a reason for the way I'd acted, but all I could think about was what Jake and I had discussed the previous night; me and my attitude. All I wanted to do was say something like "well Rob, I really don't think this is the appropriate time to discuss it...can't you see I'm trying to deal with it too? I mean, really... you want to talk about that? Come on! Don't be so self-absorbed and full of it, you asshole!"

Of course, I didn't. Instead, I thought of how I'd want to be spoken to, as Jake had demanded.

"Well Rob," I began, "I haven't all the answers you are looking for right now, but how about we meet up soon for a coffee and we can

24

chat about all that another time? Right now, I have an appointment and I'm late. Rain-check, okay?"

Before he had a chance to respond, I was gone.

As soon as I was inside the centre, I let out a sigh of relief. I was glad that little confrontation was over, but I felt good about the way I'd handled it. I actually started to feel positive, as if it was the first time I had chosen to respond calmly rather than react thoughtlessly. There's no sense in denying it: there was something to it.

After a lovely day popping around the shops and visiting the family for dinner, I returned home. I decided there was no better way to finish the day than with a glass of wine and a good movie with my feet up. As I rested on the couch and sipped on my wine, I began to feel nice and relaxed and flicked from channel to channel, searching for a good film. Bridget Jones and Mr Darcy appeared, stammering their way into each other's hearts...bingo. But no sooner was everything perfect, then 'boom!'

"Welcome to Michelle Morrissey's diary," came Jake's voice from the other end of the couch.

"Jake?! What are you doing here?" I asked, feeling very confused. "I mean I thought you only came when I was asleep?"

"I do, and you are, but forget that. More importantly, what are you doing here, on the couch, on a Friday night?" His tone became serious: "Don't tell me... are you actually in training to be the next Bridget Jones?"

He impersonated my voice in the way that's always made me roll my eyes: "Dear Diary, my best friend died, and I might as well have. I am thirty-one years old and single, and I sit in on Friday nights waiting for my Prince Charming to come through the television and sweep me gracefully off my couch, without spilling a drop of my wine."

"Well, hi there, Jake, and how are you today? How's death treating you? What's the weather like where you are? Do you have any friends on the other side? Gosh, I hope you are as pleasant to your dead friends as you are to your living ones!" I said, making my irritation clear.

"Touché," he grinned. "You haven't lost it, kiddo! So, Shelly, how are you? I know what you did today, by the by. That was very smooth with Rob. Well done."

"You mean to say you can see what I am doing all the time?" I asked, a little horrified. "Oh, that's creepy, Jake. I don't think I can cope with that, to be honest! I mean I won't be able to go to the bathroom or shower for the next twenty-one days, for God's sake."

"Chill, Shell! I have better things to be doing than watching for my best friend, who's like a sister, take a shower. Get over yourself! Besides, if I could, I'd check in on the likes of Jessica Alba or Megan Fox instead. That's not why I'm here...you can have a threesome with both of those girls, for all I care, and I wouldn't tune in for it, okay?"

"Okay," I said, warily. "So, what do you mean by 'smooth with Rob'? I thought I handled it well."

"I think you did really well, Shell, and I know the experience gave you a much better lesson than all the talking I could do in a lifetime would have, don't you think?"

"I must admit I did feel better when I handled it that way, compared to the way I used to react," I told him.

He grinned his cheeky, lovable grin. "What you're really trying to say, but don't *want* to say, is 'Jake you were so right. I don't know why I didn't listen to you when you were alive.'"

"Yes, almighty Jake; you were right. I felt better. So, what is it you are going to teach me? Enlighten me."

"Well, firstly, I want to discuss your attitude. You've got far too much of it and it's doing you no good at all."

"Wow," I said haughtily: "I wouldn't want to be sensitive now, would I?"

"Shelly trust me, you are that too. That's a whole other area we will cover another time."

"Jesus, Jake. Take it easy!"

"Look, Shell, I'm your friend, and I'm dead, so why are you taking this as a dig at you, instead of thinking 'Wow! What a wonderful opportunity to hang out with the best friend I thought I'd never see again, who loves me and cares for me and wants the best for me'?"

"You are *so* going to play that dead card regularly, aren't you?"

"I sure am."

"Okay. Sorry. I'm listening."

"Super. Let's try that again. Michelle, did I ever tell you about that old Japanese fable, *The House of a Thousand Mirrors*?"

I hated when he used my full name.

"No Jacob, I don't recall you telling me that particular story."

27

"Ok. Well, it all beganlong ago. In a small, far-away village, there was a place known as The House of a Thousand Mirrors. One day, a small happy little dog – let's call him Jake – heard of this place and decided to visit it. When he arrived, he happily bounced up the steps to the doorway of the house and looked inside with his ears up and his tail wagging as fast as it could. To his great surprise, he found himself staring at 1,000 other happy little dogs with their tails wagging just as fast as his. He smiled a great big smile and he was answered with 1,000 great big smiles just as warm and friendly as his. As he left the house, he thought to himself "what a wonderful place! I will come back and visit often!"

"In the same village, another little dog, not quite as happy as the first – let's call her Shelly – decided to visit The House of a Thousand Mirrors too. She slowly crept up the stairs and hung her head low as she looked through the doorway. When she saw 1,000 unfriendly looking dogs staring back at her, she growled at them and was horrified to see 1,000 little dogs growling back at her. As she left, she thought to herself, "what a horrible place! I will never return!""

There was a moment of silence as I thought about the message. I understood.

"I get it."

"Super!" he grinned. "True story, too!"

I was quiet as I thought about what he'd said. "You think my attitude needs some work?"

"No, Shell not at all. I think it needs less work if that makes sense."

28

"Em, no, actually it doesn't. Speak English."

"It takes a lot of work to carry an attitude like that around the place. It's much easier to just drop it. Let's look at it another way: I never really feel I try too hard with anyone. Yet, I seem far more interested and genuine than most, would you agree?"

"Yes, I suppose I do."

"Did you ever wonder why?"

"No, now that you mention it, I hadn't. Tell me why."

He paused, before blurting out "because I genuinely like people, Shell! And, because I genuinely like people, I don't have to try. It's just natural! If you force yourself upon people and try to impress them to win them over, they'll know. And if you are genuine and naturally friendly, they'll know that too. In fact, most people will gravitate towards the really genuine person. That's why I was so popular."

"And modest..." I added sarcastically. "You're saying be me. Funny, smart, talented, and ridiculously good-looking,"

"And modest," he laughed. "But, yes, Shell, and do it all with a really big smile. You need to smile more. Remember...when someone doesn't have a smile, give them yours!"

"Oh my God, Jake. I will have a pain in my face from smiling. You do know the neg-heads I work with, don't you?"

"Yes, I recall hearing you mention them a few times." Jake deadpanned. "Look at it this way; treat each person with the respect and love you would like to be treated with. You did it with Rob, so you can do it with anyone. Each and every person is an experience."

29

I am sure you are all familiar with the sensation...you know; the one that wakes you because you feel like you are falling. Well, that's what happened to me while spilling my glass of wine all over myself. Classy, I know! I moved off the couch and caught a glimpse of the time. It was 4 am and it was time to go to bed. I turned off the television and the lights and made my way to bed. Even though I didn't feel tired, I knew Jake wasn't through with me yet.

"Welcome back Shelly! Two sessions in one day...God, you really want to pack in as much as possible, don't you? You're such an eager little beaver. Seriously, though, at this rate, we will have your life turned around in no time."

I give Jake an expressionless stare.

"We were talking about Rob. Super guy! Crazy about you, Michelle, and he is everything any woman could want. After me, of course"

"God Jake," I interjected, "even in the afterlife, you are full of it!"

"Shell, like I always say, I don't think I am great, I know I am. However, I don't think I am greater than anyone else and I don't think anyone else is greater than me. There's no ego. Now back to business!

30

Shelly, have you ever read the book *Men are from Mars, Women are from Venus*?"

I took a second to search my memory.

"No. I don't think so," I said, as Jake laughed at me for even having to try to think about it.

"You definitely didn't read it because if you did, I would have known!"

"Tell me what's so great about it."

"It's one of the best books on understanding men and woman that's been written so far. That's my opinion of course. It's just so simple, logical and clever. I believe every teenager on the planet should read it. In fact, it should be on the school syllabus."

"Wow...you really like it, don't you?"

"I love that book, Shell. It inspired me to make changes to my life. And once I applied its lessons, I noticed that I had a better understanding of how women think. More importantly, I understood the difference with how men think. If you think about it Shell, all those times you had a problem in work, or in your relationships, or when you complained about your career not going anywhere, do you remember how I listened patiently? I was your shoulder to cry on, your ear to bend. I was your frustration vent!"

"I get the point, Jake. I know you were a great friend and you still are. I mean you're here to save me again, aren't you?"

"No. Shell, I'm not here to save you. I'm here to help you save yourself. All of those times that I was there for you, to quietly listen and

31

occasionally agree with you, I did because I learned that when women are worried they expect to be asked, 'are you okay honey?' They need to get the complaint out and vent, they don't necessarily want a solution to the problem there and then. They just want to vent and get it off their chest.

"I believe that this knowledge really improved my relationships, especially with Mary. Everything was easier than in my past relationships. It really helped that she had also read the book, so she had learned that men usually want a solution. However, we want to try to get it ourselves first, so we retreat into ourselves to look for one. Then, and only once we think we've got it figured out, we're ready to ask for help, which in my opinion is rare. That's why men don't want to hear, 'what's wrong?' or 'why won't you talk to me?' Or 'what are you thinking?' We need time and we'll come to you when we're ready.

"Mary used to always know when I had an issue. She never pressed me on it. She would just say, 'you'll find a solution' and she would let it go. I really loved that about her. She also learned another lesson: go to your friends to bitch and vent. She'd do that first, then come to me when she was ready for some suggestions. And that, my friend, is what you need to learn. So, today's lesson is?"

He started tapping his fingers on the coffee table, creating a drum-roll for my big reveal.

"Read *Men are from Mars, Women are from Venus*?" I responded hesitantly.

"Well, yes...that's a very good idea! But, also, understand that the greatest people who have ever lived, just like myself, knew that you can't fix anything else for anyone else until you fix yourself."

"Ha-ha Jake, you are so funny. You're so modest!"

"Seriously! Some of the greatest people who have ever lived have said 'you should work more on yourself than you do your job.' Shelly, read books that teach you how to be your best. Listen to audiobooks, go to seminars, and hang out with people who are good at living. Success leaves clues. Are you with me?"

"Yes, I am. I agree with you about working on ourselves. I mean nobody really teaches us how to use our mind, and if you think about it, we spend our whole life using it don't we?"

"Exactly! You're beginning to see the importance of investing in yourself and how you think! Buddha said 'your world is comprised of you and of your thoughts: the wise man controls his thoughts.'"

"That one lesson taught me to live a much happier life, and you deserve to see and feel that same positive difference in your life. I just want you to be happy."

"I know Jake, and I want that too. I'll buy the book first thing in the morning."

"I have a better idea Shell. Swing by my place tomorrow and take my copy and while you are at it, check out my collection of books and, see if anything else tickles your fancy."

"I was going to call to Sam and your mum anyway to hang out."

33

Samantha is Jake's younger sister but she is also like a little sister to me. Jake's mum, Mary, well...she's like another mother.

He smiled at me.

"I want to leave you with an analogy I learned many years ago. In life, you should be like the good gardener. What does a good gardener do?"

I paused to think before answering. I'd always hated quizzes.

"He plucks the weeds?"

"What else?"

"He waters the flowers."

"Yes, good. What else?"

"Ummm...he...I don't know Jake! I'm not much of a gardener!"

"Come on Shell, just guess."

"He plants flowers."

"Exactly! The good gardener plants the flowers, waters the flowers and pulls up the weeds. Your mind is like a garden, and you're the gardener. The weeds are your negative thoughts, all your worries and stresses, and the flowers are your positive thoughts. The flowers are your wishes and dreams. A good gardener knows that he must plant the seeds to get the flowers and he knows he must water them for them to grow. Are you with me?"

"Totally! I'm all ears."

"Okay, super! So the gardener also knows that the weeds will grow no matter what, right?"

I nodded in agreement.

34

"So he has to watch out and catch them early before they do any damage. He also knows that the more regularly he plucks them, the less quickly they will grow back. Just like our negative thoughts. We have to cultivate our thoughts. We have to design our ideal garden."

"I love that, Jake. I love the whole idea. It makes so much sense! This stuff should definitely be taught in schools."

"I know!" he agreed. "I'm glad you like it. So, it's time again. Shelly, put it to practice. Till next time, kiddo."

He turned to leave, and I woke up to the sun shining in the window.

*Chapter 4 - Sleep 4*

*Saturday, October 26th*

It was a sunny Saturday morning. I got up, showered and got ready to enjoy the day. Even though I slept half the night on the couch, I still felt really good, just as Jake had promised. After breakfast, I made my way to the Lawlor household. Because it was such a nice day, I decide to walk. It was beautiful; dry, fresh and sunny. The autumn leaves had fallen along the roadside and footpath and I kicked through them as I walked. I started to think about the advice Jake had given me, and as I approached the Lawlor house, I repeated the mantra: "Be the good gardener."

I gently tapped on the back door as I opened it, and called out as I walked into the kitchen.

"Hello? Anybody home?"

Our families had been close for a long time. Jake's mum and my mum are both nurses in the local hospital and had worked together for over 25 years.

Both families had three children each, and all around the same ages. Jake was the middle child in his family at just 33, with an older brother Michael, 35, and younger sister Sam, who was 27. I am the middle in my family at 31 with an older sister Cara, 34, and a younger sister Eve who's 25. We were a gang, we four girls and two boys. We were all brothers and sisters.

I heard Mary's voice calling from upstairs; "Up here, Shell."

I walked up the stairs toward Jake's room and Sam popped her head around the door. I greeted the girls with hugs and kisses and asked them how they were doing. Mary fussed and bustled.

"Not as well as you by the looks of it! What did you have for breakfast?"

I laughed awkwardly as I realised that nobody else is getting these visits from Jake, and nobody knows that Jake is visiting me in my sleep either. They had no reason to be as upbeat as me. They were still in mourning. I knew I had to explain why I was so cheery,

"Oh, I am just feeling a bit better today. Probably because I got a good night's sleep. Really, though, I'm just taking it day by day. I think that's what Jake would do, don't you?"

"Hell yes!" Sam explained. "Guru Jake!" We all laughed because it was true.

"If it were him here and one of us were gone, he would be all philosophical about it. 'We are all energy and energy can't be created or destroyed' or something like that!"

Sam lay back on Jake's bed, and we couldn't help but laugh at her impersonation of her big brother.

"You're on the ball!" I said. "He would totally have said that, and that's why we loved him and, more importantly, that's why he was so

37

happy all the time. It was his way of looking at things that really did it." As I said those words, I felt like I understood him more.

Mary sat on the bed next to Sam and I and she placed a hand on each of us, "Girls, I have done lots of things in my life I wish I had done differently and some of them made things tougher for all of us, I know that. But it made us stronger. Jake helped me to see that a long time ago."

She started to cry and we hugged her from either side.

"Jake helped me feel and see more joy in my life. I know that if I focus on being happy and positive, in a way I'll always have him around. He was so full of life and love. And Shelly, I meant to say it to you after the funeral, we really appreciated you doing the eulogy. It was beautiful and he would have liked your words."

"Thanks, Mary," I murmured.

"I'm sure he heard them."

"I am too," I said with a little internal smile. She had no idea how right she was. Mary gestured around at the mess in the room.

"Well, we better get some of these clothes into bags, girls. Shelly, if there is anything that you would like to take as a keepsake, please do. I know Jake would want that."

"Ah thanks, Mary. Actually, there were one or two books Jake had mentioned to me recently that he said were very good. If that's okay, can I take a few books?"

"Work away, love."

38

Mary started to go through Jake's wardrobes as I looked through the bookshelves. I spotted *Men are from Mars, Women are from Venus* and Sam caught my eye as I picked it up.

"Oh," she said with a grin; "the relationship bible."

"Excuse me?" I said, slightly puzzled.

"That's what Jake used to call that book. It's actually really good. Jake got it for me as part of my 21$^{st}$ birthday present and he made me read it and then tested me after."

"Did you find it useful?"

"Shelly, you have met me?! Yeah! " she replied confidently.

I looked at Sam and realised that there, right in front of me, was a girl all the guys wanted to get with, and who all the girls wanted to be. Sam had her pick of men and always seemed to be going on dates or in a relationship, and the funny thing was, she was always happy in those relationships. Sam always had fun, and even if they were short relationships, they were sweet. She had loads of male as well as female friends and she gelled well with all of them.

"Now that I think about it, yeah. Sam you do seem to be good at relationships. Well, getting into them anyway," I said, mocking her gently.

"I am good at getting them and I am good in them!" she protested. "The only reason I haven't had a long-term relationship is because I'm in the experience stage of my life, that's all!"

"Oh, is that what you call it?" I said cheekily.

"Well, Shell, when I was just a teenager Jake told me to just have fun and not to get too carried away with anybody but myself. When I hit 21 and he gave me the book, he asked me if that had been good advice. Well, it was. So he gave me the book with a little note inside. He called it his 'second snippet'. It was more relationship advice."

"What did the note say?"

"That's actually my copy," she said, gesturing to the paperback in my hands. "You can see for yourself."

I opened the book and started to read what Jake had written.

"*To my darling sister Sam, on your 21st birthday.*

*Here is lesson No. 2 on the topic of relationships! The next few years of your life are like going to college. The subject is successful relationships and the qualifications are as follows: Year 1: Certificate; Years 2-3: Diploma; Year 4: Degree; Year 6: Masters; Year 8; PhD.*

*"Choose how long you want to study and how much of an expert you want to become. But remember: knowledge is only potential power. You have to use it for it to be powerful. When you meet a wonderful person that you feel that connection with; someone you can see clearly you have a future with, take a little more time before jumping into marriage. If you are happy and it's meant to be, then stay happy and wait for a little while longer.*

*We don't get older; we get better.*

*Love always,*

*Jake xxx*"

Sam watched me reading until I got to the end.

"See? So I'm just enjoying the experience at the moment. I couldn't imagine getting married before 30 anyway," she said with great certainty in her voice.

A voice shouted out from downstairs.

"Anybody home?"

It was my Mum and my sisters, Eve and Cara. Cara had come home from Canada for the funeral.

Mary made her way downstairs and called behind her to Sam and me.

"Come on girls, let's have a cuppa."

I glimpsed through the other books and spotted one or two more books that Jake had mentioned at one time or another. As Sam was going out the door, she turned around and tapped me on the arm.

"Shelly take whatever books you like, but I recommend you take at least one DVD. Trust me, I know you well enough to know you were never the most avid reader, but you are very visual."

"Okay Sam, thanks. So, any recommendations?"

Sam looked at the selection of DVDs and picked one out straight away; "*The Peaceful Warrior*, hun. Definitely."

"Super, thanks. Hang on...what do you mean by 'visual'?"

She looked at me and smiled.

"Seriously Shell, are you sure you hung around with my brother? Look take that N.L.P book next to the DVD that will explain it to you."

41

Sam ran down stairs and left me to make my selection of books. The girls were in the kitchen, chatting. I looked around Jake's room, taking it all in. The shelves of books were nearly floor to ceiling taking up an entire wall. I grabbed one or two more and some DVDs and made my way towards the door, noticing something I had never seen before, a quote on the wall above Jake's bed, written in calligraphy:

*"When I was five years old my mother always told me that happiness was the key to life.*

*When I went to school, they asked me what I wanted to be when I grew up.*

*I wrote down 'Happy.'*

*They told me I didn't understand the assignment, and I told them they didn't understand life."*

*John Lennon*

I made my way downstairs, smiling. I felt like I was really starting to see the world with new eyes and it felt good.

I became excited at the idea of speaking to Jake again that night. I think I even considered going for a nap when I got home. I walked into the kitchen and the girls are gathered around the table chatting and drinking tea.

Sam and Eve were huddled together as if attached at the hip. They'd been like that most of their lives, and it reminded me of Jake and myself at their age. Sam had far better communication skills than my own sister. Even though the girls were the best of friends – close in age, both good looking and both nice girls – Sam seemed more confident and carefree than Eve had ever been. I sat down to join them and I looked closely at them. The more I observed, the more I saw the reasons why they are so different.

Eve never needed to work when she was going school, as our parents had wanted us to focus on our educations. Sam, on the other hand, had worked in a restaurant through school, and bars through college, and she was far more approachable than Eve was. They were a lot like Jake and me. Jake had also worked in restaurants and bars when he was younger, while I hadn't worked until after college.

"Hello, Shelly. Earth calling Shelly," my sister Cara joked as she tried to get my attention. "Seeing as you are off for the week, do you think you could drop me to the airport on Monday morning, please?"

"Yeah, sure I will. No problem."

We continued chatting for a bit, we talked about Cara's new life in Canada with her baby, Samhain, and her husband, Kevin. She told us all about Samhain and how he is starting to become such a character now.

"He is such a good child, but he's not very interested in going to bed at night at the moment. Like most children, I suppose!"

That got the mothers talking about when we were all small and the mischief we got up to. Mum recalled Cara playing hide and seek with Eve and me once when I was nowhere to be found for about a half hour.

"I was frantic!" she said dramatically. "I had called to all the neighbours and there were about ten people out looking for you. I remember them all over the road and in the house shouting 'Michelle!

43

Stop hiding! The game is over!' Eventually one of the neighbours randomly looked in one of their kitchen presses, and there was my little Goldilocks, curled up in a ball, fast asleep and none the wiser to all the drama and panic that was going on around her."

We laughed as we reminisced and before we knew it, it was lunchtime. We decided we'd go to the pub to grab a bite to eat. Lunch turned into drinks, drinks turned into dinner, and dinner turned into more drinks. At 11 pm, Dad and Jake's brother Michael collected our drunken posse, corralling us into their cars. I was dropped off after Mum and the girls and the last thing I remember hearing as I drifted off to sleep was the song *Galileo* again. A familiar voice was singing along.

"Who puts the rainbow in the sky? Who lights the stars at night?"

I turned my head and realised I was in the back of Dad's car, with Jake singing next to me.

"Jake? What happened?!"

"Well Shelly, you and the rest of the girls got very drunk. Then, as usual, your dad picked you and your sisters up and dropped them home and now he is escorting you home. You've fallen into one of your trademark drunken comas, hence why we are in the back of his car while he drives! Don't worry, he can't hear us. At this rate, you will have used up all your sleeps in no time."

The thought made me sad again. I knew we'd have to say goodbye for good sometime soon.

44

"What's the deal with 21 sleeps anyway? Why 21? I mean, why would you pick that random number?"

"It's not random!" he replied. "It's actually quite a significant number. However, it doesn't account for the possibility that you would be falling asleep more than once a day. To be honest, I sort of overlooked that one. Be that as it may, changes that you start to make in your life should always be done for a minimum of 21 days. That's how long it takes to make or break a habit. In the words of Aristotle, 'We are what we repeatedly do.' In which case you could be an alcoholic or a narcoleptic!"

"Hardly," I objected, "but I guess that makes sense. In fact, I think I remember you and Rob doing something like that before. You did some sort of twenty-one somethings for twenty-one days for charity a few years back?"

"Oh yes, we did! It was a challenge where we did twenty-one burpees, twenty-one times per day for twenty-one days to raise money for the Hospice. We got super fit doing them!"

"What on earth," I slurred, "is a burpee?!"

Jake looked at me in bemusement.

"You do a knees to chest jump, into a squat and then jump back into a push-up and then repeat the process. We did something like four hundred and forty a day. It was over nine thousand burpees by the end of the twenty-one days. Ouch."

"Shell? Shell, wake up my love." I think I half woke as Dad nudged me gently,

"Time to go home to bed, sweetheart."

45

"Okay Dad, thanks for bringing me home."

I felt like I was still asleep and not 100% in control of my body. Dad walked alongside me into the house. I told him I was fine. "Go on away home," I told him. "I'm ok, I promise. I am going to go to bed now to chat to Jake, so no need to worry."

Dad ignored my drunken comment and practically carried me upstairs to bed. I was still half asleep and I kept talking to Jake as if it was a normal situation, "Jake, look how good my dad is. Good old Gary. Gary, Gary, Gary. Gary the great. You the man, Dad."

Luckily, Gary the Great didn't pay me too much attention. He placed me on my bed, threw the blanket over me and turned off the light. "Night night, sweetheart, sleep well."

As he was leaving my bedroom, I mumbled, "Jake say bye to dad."

By that time dad was already down the stairs and in the process of locking the front door.

"Good job Shelly, now your dad thinks you're just plain crazy."

I felt very confused.

"You were just half asleep, half awake and you spoke to your dad and me at the same time, as if it was normal."

"I did?"

"Well, you asked me to say goodbye as he was leaving."

There was a pause and I burst out laughing. Then after a short time, Jake bursts out laughing too.

"Oh! Oh, Jake. Does that mean I used a sleep or not?"

"Technically no. You were still half asleep, so lucky for you! Okay, now back to business. So, as I was saying earlier about the twelve to twenty-one days, it's not so much the time that it takes as much as it is the consistency that makes something a habit. The best of the best, from Bruce Lee to The Beatles, became the best because they were consistent. Ten thousand hours of practice, so they say. Remember what I said the other night, Shelly?"

"Success leaves clues?" I replied hesitantly.

"Yes! Very good. If you were to look at your life, where do you think you might have put in 10,000 hours at anything?"

I start to think about the question.

"Does thinking hurt?" Jake asked smartly.

I don't even answer. I disregard his jibe and kept thinking.

"I suppose piano. I have definitely played ten thousand hours of piano."

"Perfect example, and would you consider yourself good at it?"

"I suppose so."

"What? You suppose? Right, make a mental note that next time we meet we need to discuss confidence."

"Well okay Jake, yes. Yes, I am good."

"Try again."

"Okay, Jake. I am excellent at the piano."

"Very good Shell, so now that you know you can only get better at something the more you do it, what would you like to test it out on?"

"What do you mean?"

47

"I mean you should pick something to work on, like an area of your life that you would like to improve. Decide what you would like to accomplish or improve in that area and give yourself a time-frame. In the words of Napoleon Hill 'A Goal is a dream with a deadline.'

"Do you remember when you were learning how to drive?"

I could tell the question would no doubt lead to an analogy or a story of some description.

"Well, yeah, kind of," I told him and waited for him to get to the point.

"Right, do you remember how difficult it was at times? How you struggled to remember what to do next? There were even times when you would conk out in the middle of the road. Sometimes you would grind the gears and sometimes you would rev the engine and..."

"Okay. Okay, Jake. Yes. What's your point?"

"Well, did you get out of the car when it conked and say, 'I give up'? Did you ever walk away and leave the car in the middle of the road?"

"No. But only because Dad wouldn't leave me!"

"No, you didn't. You got back in and you tried again and you kept going until eventually, you were able to drive, correct?"

"Yes, you are right. I didn't give up, I kept going. I can drive."

"Okay, now, explain to me how to drive a car, Shelly."

"Well...uh...you start the engine...and then you put the car into gear and, oh, you check the mirrors," I was really struggling to explain. "Then you, then you put your foot on the accelerator, and, uh...then..."

48

"Right Shell, stop! Do you, maybe, think perhaps that you would have started the car quicker than you can explain how to start the car?"

"Definitely."

"So don't you maybe think that the hardest part of learning most things is the thinking part? Getting it into your head?"

"I suppose."

"It is because once it becomes a habit you no longer need to think so much about it. It's autopilot, and the part that makes things happen is the action; the thinking is no longer necessary. In fact, as you can see, if anything, it's the thinking that makes it harder."

"You're right," I agreed. "It does. I know I could go and drive my car and I wouldn't think at all about how. I just do it. I must admit I never thought it would be difficult to explain it but it is. It's definitely easier to just do it."

"That's it exactly. I don't think you need to learn anymore. If you get that, then that's everything."

"Really?!" I asked in surprise.

"No, Shelly. That's not all. I'm kidding with you. But it *is* very important, because if you get that idea, then it can be applied to most areas of your life. Not only is that not all, but we're only getting started!"

"What do you mean, Jake? Have you got a schedule laid out for me or something?"

"Well, yes. Kind of. That's the idea, anyway. I suppose I can give you a sneak preview of what's to come." I sat up in the bed, all ears.

49

"Like I told you, I will be coming to you for 21 sleeps. We have had four sleeps so far and I feel like we've laid some good foundations. Over the days to come, we will discuss some of the most basic and fundamental lessons a person can learn to help improve their life."

"Such as?"

"How to improve your health, your fitness and your mindset. Oh, and we'll have to talk about starting your bucket list!"

"That's things to do before you die?"

"Yes, but you're missing the point: it's things to do while you are alive. Look at me! I'm dead and I made that list while I was alive and I did lots because of it. Not everything, but enough to have had some great experiences."

"Fair point. I know you did loads and a bucket list helped. I definitely need to do one."

"I also think over the next while it would be nice to work on learning to let go and never giving up, and we'll throw in some giving and gratitude just for fun!"

"Sounds good Batman. I'm getting excited!"

"Good to know, Robin. So, should we make our way to the Batpoles?"

I laughed at the thought of us running around in costume as Batman and Robin...a Dynamic Duo if ever there was one.

"Remember," Jake told me, serious again: "Rome wasn't built in a day but a bit of it was." Jake's laugh was the last thing I heard until I woke to the familiar sound of rain hitting my window.

As I lay in bed listening to the rain, I noticed how good I felt, considering the amount I'd had to drink the previous day. Jake wasn't kidding with the feeling good when I wake deal. Sweet! I stretched out on the bed, getting ready to hop out of it, and my phone rang.

"Top of the morning to you!" I answered enthusiastically.

"Jesus, Shell, how are you so full of beans?"

It was my sister, Eve.

"I guess I'm just more experienced than you," I replied smugly.

"Experience was Mum and Mary not drinking spirits with us and knowing when to stop! I'm dying with the hangover from hell! No thanks to you and those JD and Cokes."

"Nobody forced you to drink them, Evie. Besides, don't you think you are old enough to take responsibility for your own hangover?"

She didn't take too kindly to that.

"Oh my God, Shell, you win. I'm just not able this morning. My brain is mush. I'm calling because we thought you might want to spend some quality time with your little sis and big sis; while we have her around. Maybe breakfast, to start? You can drive, seeing as you're in such flying form."

"No problem! I'll pick you up in half an hour, okay?"

51

"Perfect! See you then."

I jumped out of bed, something I don't usually do, had a quick shower, got dressed and headed off. As I approached my parents' house, I beeped the horn and girls appeared at the door looking worse for wear. "Feeling a little rough around the edges?" I giggled.

"What the hell! Are you not hungover?" demanded Cara; "we're dying!"

"Yeah!" adds Eve. "Highly suspicious. I mean, you're always the one in a sad state the morning after. What miracle drug have you taken? I want some."

I laughed at their envy, and then I changed the subject.

"Let's go get some breakfast. Where to?"

"The Coffee Dock," Eve said before Cara had even had a chance to speak. "I really want bacon and eggs on sourdough. Can we go there?" I can tell when Eve has made up her mind. When she knows what she wants, she won't stop until she gets it. Cara didn't have the energy to offer an alternative. Next stop, Coffee Dock.

As I drove I started to think about the allegory Jake had discussed, and his philosophical musings about driving a car, and how over-thinking can interfere with the action. About halfway there, I realised that I was thinking too much and distracting myself and that if I kept it up I might end up having an accident.

After breakfast we decided to have a little retail therapy, so we made our way to the city for a spot of shopping. I bought Cara's little boy Samhain a birthday present, as we were just a month away from his first

52

after lots of tossing and

birthday celeb

there was Jake.

to head home

"What did you

for Cara bef

"Oh my God, J

arrived hom

moving!"

dinner. The

I couldn't wait to

enthusiastically.

finished a

"I think my favou

time to g

pond and, then, Dan runs

good ma

mind.' Socrates responds,

though

clever."

Queen

"I'm glad you like

favourites. I must have watc

had b

sisterly, family hangout day.

saw t

"It was great, but I

new

"What I really want

different?"

to I

"Well, I think I am s

tha

people a little differently. I sup

th

first time if that makes sense?"

v

"It makes perfect ser

i

keep happening. It's a great op

you, but also to become more p

to be doing what you're doing."

rning, I think I must have just nodded off, and

hink?"

ke I loved it! It's just so meaningful and

talk about it, and I sat up in the bed very

ite bit is when Socrates pushes Dan into the
fter him screaming at him, 'you are out of your
know. It's taken me a lifetime.' It's just so

it!" he said with a smile. "It's one of my
ed it ten times. I noticed you had a little
low did that go?"
am sure you know all about it anyway."
to know is, what have you noticed that's

arting to observe my family and other
ose I feel as if I am seeing them for the

se, and now that you are aware of it, it will
ortunity to really learn from those around
resent. It's key to be where you are and

I found that a little confusing. "What do you mean?" I had to ask. "You've kind of lost me there."

"Okay...imagine you are hanging out with a friend, say Laura from the band. Let's say Laura has had a bad day and she's unloading her stresses on you. She's talking, talking, talking, and you're zoning in and zoning out. So one minute you're listening, then the next minute you start thinking of other things like what you wanted to say next, or 'did I turn off my hair straightener?' or 'what time is my appointment tomorrow?' Does that sound familiar?"

"Yeah. It does, actually."

"There are moments between talking and listening, and those are the moments when you're thinking. The worst part of that is when you're having those thoughts, you might as well not be there with your friend. In fact, you're never really with someone when you are thinking of someone or something else."

"Jake that's just like *The Peaceful Warrior*. I totally do that! Oh, my God, I feel awful. But, that means people do that to me too, yeah?"

"Of course! But other people are not your responsibility. You are responsible for you and the way you control your thoughts and the way you pay attention to people. Last night you had a real 'in the moment' experience with your Mum and Dad. You watched them, you listened to them and, most importantly, you were completely within the experience. That's being in the moment, Shelly. That's what every experience should be. That's what you should be doing every moment of the day, or as much as you possibly can."

55

"So you are telling me to pay more attention to everything going on around me all the time?"

"Yes. It's about hearing, seeing, feeling, tasting and smelling everything that's going on at every moment. Remember there's never nothing going on."

I was beginning to understand what Jake was saying.

"I can see what you mean," I told him. "Live in the moment."

"Exactly. It's like when you're singing. I can't tell you how many times I've watched you and heard you when you sing and I can feel the passion coming from you with every word. I can always tell you're in that moment, whether you are singing someone else's song or one of your own. I know that's when you are in the flow. It's obvious to everyone."

"Whatever, Jake! Don't go all soft on me."

"Michelle, I am giving you a compliment! When someone gives you a compliment, you could at least have the good decency to accept it."

"Then thanks, I suppose."

"What I really mean is that you can't be in your head, and at the same time out in the world doing something properly in the moment. Do you not agree? If you were singing and thinking of other things you would probably forget words or sing offbeat, wouldn't you?"

"I see your point," I admitted.

"I can remember a scene from that movie you took me to see when Mary and I split up. Forgetting...something?" He furrowed his brow trying to think of it, but I know the one he meant,

"*Forgetting Sarah Marshall.*"

56

"Right! That's the one. Well, there's a scene when Mila Kunis's character says 'Get out of your head, it's nice out here.' I love that line. It just says it all."

"I don't remember her saying that but it's a good one."

"Also, a simple tip I learned years ago, is to stamp your feet on the ground, to remind yourself where you are. Just take it all on board, Shell, and remember: the worst that can happen is that it will improve your life."

"I will start first thing in the morning, Jake."

As soon as I said that, I remembered why I'd set my alarm clock nice and early. "Cara is going back to Canada tomorrow," I told him with a note of sadness in my voice. "I'll miss her."

"I know you will. Cara's great. She's always had a really good outlook on life, and I learned a lot from her."

I'm surprised to hear Jake say that about her.

"She is quite a character," he continued. "She's always been the sporty one in your family. She knows all about being in the flow; it's a natural part of playing sport. She knows all about it, without realising it."

"Yeah. She's a good big sister. She's always so understanding and full of good advice. She's the only one of the three of us that never holds a grudge!"

"Exactly, Shell. She lives in the now and doesn't carry past issues. In fact, I think Cara is like that because she was that bit older than us when all the hassle with my Dad was happening. I think she learned a lot from seeing what we all went through."

57

"I can imagine that she did see a lot of the stuff you have told me about over the years. She and Michael were joined at the hip, kinda like you and me."

"Yeah they were and I think they still have a great relationship, after all, he introduced her to Kevin."

"True."

"It's time for me to go, Shell. It's time for you to go pick up your sister and make sure she gets to the airport safely. I'll see you tomorrow night, and until then, try to stay out of your head."

As I was about to promise Jake that I'd try, my alarm went off and jolted me awake. It was 6 am. I jumped out of bed and stretched with a content sigh. "Life isn't half bad," I said to myself. I got dressed, brushed my teeth and threw cold water on my face to freshen up. I walked downstairs to the kitchen. On my way, I saw the postman approaching the house. He seemed to be almost skipping along. I opened the door and walk outside to greet him.

"Good morning."

"Good morning, Miss Morrissey," he replied as he passed me my mail. "Quite unusual to see you up and about at this time of the morning!"

"I know," I told him, "but I have to drop my sister to the airport; early flight, you know."

"Oh this is the best time of the day," he replied with a grin. "I always feel like I have the world to myself for the first few hours of the day. It's so peaceful and quiet."

"I bet it is! Please, call me Shelly. And...I'm sorry, you've been my postman for years and I've never asked...what's your name?"

"Pat," he said with a cheeky grin.

I raised an eyebrow.

"Seriously? Postman Pat?"

"No," he laughed, "but it was worth it to see your reaction. My name's Troy."

"Well nice to meet you, Troy."

"Nice to meet you, Shelly," he smiled as he reached out to shake my hand.

"You must really love your work," I told him. "You seem to be very happy for so early in the morning."

"I have the best job in the world," he beamed. "I start at 6 am and I finish at 2 pm. I have a lovely route and I've had it for 20 years. I get to be out and about at the best time of the day, and then I get home to spend time with my wife and family in the evening. It's great. Is your sister Cara back off to Canada today then?"

"Yes, she is. Do you know her?"

"I sure do. She's the sporty one! Back when she was training, she used to be up for a run every morning at six o'clock. I always liked her. She is a very pleasant girl and a real morning person too. We're rare!"

I took a look around and there's nobody around except he and I.

"I can see that!" I agreed.

"Your friend Jake was the same. He was a lovely chap...I was very sad to hear the news," he said with a sombre tone. "You spoke so well at his funeral. Well done."

I know my face betrayed my surprise.

"Oh, you were there?"

"Oh God yes! Everyone in the town knew Jake. He was one in a million. I remember when my little girl Amelie was born nine years ago, he was one of the first to congratulate me. He even sent my wife flowers and got me a round of drinks in Gallagher's, back when he worked there. I saw him every morning for the last 10 years out running or cycling regardless of the weather. His training was like my job. It didn't matter the weather, he turned up."

His perspective on Jake made me happy, but time was up.

"Well Troy, it's been lovely chatting with you but I'd better get going or I'll be late."

"Lovely chatting to you too, Shelly. Have a good day, and you never know; I might see you another morning."

"I wouldn't put money on it!" I laughed. "I'm not a morning person like you and Cara and Jake!"

Troy looked at me with a smile.

"Jake used to say, 'I am not a morning person, I am an all–day person!' I thought that was very clever. So, you never know, Shelly."

"Yeah, that sounds like Jake. See ya, Troy."

"Bye bye, Shelly. Have a good day!"

As I approached the house I spotted Cara's suitcase at the front door, Cara and Eve came out the door, with Mum and Dad behind them still in their pyjamas.

I rolled down the car window.

"Good morning, family!"

"Morning hun," Mum shouted. Eve, still half asleep, just about mumbled "Hey."

Dad carried Cara's suitcase to the car and into the boot as Cara sat in. She looked at me, still sleepy, and asked how I was.

"Super, thanks!" I answered. "And you? Are we good to go?"

"We sure are!"

As we drove off, the family waved and shouted.

"Bye, Cara! Love you! Safe home!"

Cara waved and shouted out the window. "Love you too! Bye!"

"Well we are on schedule," I told her. "Your flight isn't until 9 am. Do you want to grab breakfast after you check in?"

"Yeah. That would be great," she said.

Cara turned away from the window and looked at me with her head tilted and a confused expression on her face.

"This is a surprise. I thought you were going to drop me off at the door and go straight back home to bed!"

I couldn't help but laugh.

"Yeah, well...I'm up now, so I might as well keep you company...but only because I feel sorry for you!"

"Thanks!" she laughed. "Well since you feel sorry for me, breakfast is your treat."

We arrived at the airport, Cara checked in and in no time at all, we were sitting down having breakfast.

"Oh. I forgot to tell you Troy the postman was asking for you."

"Oh my God, I haven't seen him in years. Although I think he was at the funeral."

"He was. He told me this morning."

"He's a nice man. He's been doing that route for years."

"He has. 20 of them."

"Wow Shelly!" she said with genuine surprise: "It's unusual for you to be so interested in people you don't know. Did he tell you his life story?"

"No, just a few bits. Nice man, great attitude."

"Yes, he is," Cara agreed, but I could tell she was still a little surprised. She looked me in the eye and took a deep breath.

"How are you holding up, Shell? I mean...you know. With everything that's happened."

"I'm actually really good," I told her, even though I knew she was sceptical. "I feel a new lease of life to be honest. I really want to live

62

a happier and healthier life. I suppose Jake's passing has given me a greater appreciation of things. Do you know what I mean?"

"Yes, I do. And that's great, Shell, but just be aware it's okay to mourn. That's all part of the healing process too."

I knew she was right, and I knew she was worried about me.

"Cara, can I ask you something?"

"You can ask me anything."

"Well, you know when you were growing up? Did you see a lot of what went on in the Lawlor's family with their dad?"

"I suppose I saw enough. Mum and Dad didn't want us to be exposed to it. But I do remember times when Mary and the kids would stay at our place, and times when Dad had to go over to their house to calm Pat down."

This was news to me.

"What was he like?"

"Oh, he was a demon! I was petrified of him; we all were. He was a scary man when he was mad. I remember one time we were all there playing and he got into a temper. He'd been drinking, of course. I saw him throw the kitchen table through the kitchen window. Mary bought all of us upstairs into one of the bedrooms and told us to play camp. I think she must have called Mum and Dad. They came over and took us all to our house. Crazy stuff! He was like The Hulk. I don't know how Mary put up with it for as long as she did."

It was very sad to think about. After a few moment's silence, I asked the obvious question.

"Do you think it affected Jake's life?"

"Yes, I do. It had to have. And Michael's; maybe Sam, but not as much. She was a little younger. I believe it made them better people because they choose not to be like him. Michael is one of my best friends and one of the most kind, caring men I know. He is a gentleman, and I know there isn't a bad bone in his body. Jake was like a little brother to me and he was probably one of my favourite people in the world. I loved everything about him. He was caring and kind, smart, fun...interesting and wise beyond his years. If that boy wrote a book on how to be happy, it would be a number-one best seller! After his father died, I think he just decided that life is for living and he enjoyed every second of it.

"I plan on doing the same," she continued. "Jake's death has inspired me to enjoy the life I have and not take a moment for granted. He always said 'we are here for a good time, not a long time.' I liked that idea." It made me happy to see her beaming smile while she remembered Jake.

"I know what you mean," I said. "I...I feel like he's still here, you know? He's still here, guiding me. So, if you feel like he's guiding you too, then go with it..."

We sat there in silence for a few minutes, sipping coffees and remembering things in our own ways. I was keeping a close eye on the clock and became acutely aware of passing time.

"When will ye be coming home again?" I asked, out of nowhere.

"Ha!" Cara exclaimed, "More like, when will you be coming to visit?"

"Good question! I suppose I could take a few weeks in the summer."

"That would be great!" she smiled. "Sonya is coming out to visit in June, once the schools are done for summer holidays. Why don't you travel with her? There is plenty of room in our place. We have three bedrooms, and you get on with Sonya right?"

Sonya was one of Cara's oldest friends. I'd known her since I was very young.

"Yeah, we get on great."

"So ye could share a room. And you'd be company for each other on the journey over."

"That sounds like a plan. In fact, I am going to start planning that soon. I will contact Sonya and suss things out. How is she?"

"She's great! Apparently, she was on television here recently. There was a documentary about her studio. Did you see it?"

"No, I didn't," I replied. I hadn't even heard about it. "I definitely have to call her now, we have loads to catch up on! Awesome! I'm going to Canada!" That was that; a plan had been made. I wouldn't be allowed to forget it. Cara smiled warmly and glanced up at the clock.

"I'd better get going for my gate," she sighed, and we got up and walked towards the long queue for security.

"I love you, Shelly," she said with a smile as she wrapped her arms around me and pulled me into a bear hug.

65

"Love you too!" I murmured as I squeezed her. "Text me when you arrive home ok?"

"I will. Mind yourself, and you have my number if you need to chat anytime."

"Thanks. I know. And I'll see you in June," I grinned before we let go of each other and she made her way towards the metal detector.

I watched until she was gone around the corner into Departures, then headed back to my car. It was only 8.30am, and as I walked along I wondered what I would do for the day. I finally decided to call one of the few people I knew were guaranteed to be up at this time of the morning. I pulled out my phone and dialled the number from memory.

"Hello, Rob."

"Oh, hey Shelly. To what do I owe the pleasure?"

"Well, I was just wondering if you want to meet up for a coffee."

"Now?"

"Yeah, sure, if you're free."

"Okay, where?"

"Great! Meet you at the Coffee Dock in an hour?"

"See you then."

"Super," I said. "See you then"

I hung up the phone, hopped into my car and headed straight for the Coffee Dock. When I got there, Rob was sitting in the corner. He was wearing a suit and looked quite handsome. I took my time as I made my way towards where he was sitting, thinking about how our relationship used to be, and I felt a little sad about how I had ended it. Finally, I sat down across from him.

"You're looking very suave this morning!"

He grinned and made a show of straightening his tie.

"I have an appointment at the bank after this."

"Oh, really?" I think he could tell I was genuinely interested.

"Yeah, I'm looking to expand the gym and I was supposed to meet with the bank manager last week, but with all that has happened I had to reschedule."

"Oh, that's fabulous, Rob! Well done and best of luck."

"Thanks! So...how are you keeping?"

"I'm good, thanks. I just dropped Cara to the airport and thought I would chance it and see if you were free for that cuppa and catch-up."

"What did you want to talk about?" he asked. I think he might have been a little suspicious.

"I suppose I was hoping you and I could start over as friends. If you're cool with that?"

He paused.

"I don't know," he answered slowly. "I'm really not sure how I feel at the moment."

I hadn't been expecting that.

"What do you mean?" I asked.

"It's not that I don't want to be friends," he answered, "but I've lost a friend too, you know? And I lost you, too. I was just starting to get on with things and there you were, back in my life again. I don't know how I feel about that. I mean...I don't think I can be friends. I have feelings, Shelly. I need to move on. I can't do that and be friends with you."

I looked at him, stunned. I hadn't been prepared to hear that at all.

The best I could manage was a weak "Oh." I knew he needed to hear more than that, so I took a breath and started again. "I hope someday we can be friends, and you know I'll always care for you. You're a wonderful guy. I really want you to be happy." We sat there awkwardly, our eyes downcast. I told him that I had to go. As I got up to leave, Rob grabbed my arm gently.

"Shelly, tell me...I really need to know: is there any chance for us?"

I looked him straight in the eyes. He needed to hear the truth. "No. We were done when I ended it. We just weren't meant to be. It's time for you to move on. Find someone who deserves you." I don't know why, but I leant over and hugged him goodbye. Neither of us said another word.

As I left the Coffee Dock I felt a little upset, but I was glad I'd met with him. I knew that was important for him to move on, and as hard as it might have been, this was the only way. It was closure.

I hadn't been there long enough to get a coffee, so I decided to go home to have a cuppa and to start reading one of Jake's books. After reading for what seemed like the whole day, I looked at the clock. It was 10 pm. I felt tired enough to go to bed. Besides, I had been up since 6 am so it made sense to have an early night. I turned off the lights, locked the doors and made my way upstairs to bed. No sooner had I lain down than I was fast asleep.

"Early to bed and early to rise makes a girl healthy, wealthy and wise," Jake's voice sang to me.

"Yeah, I've heard that one before," I told him. "Do you actually believe that?"

"Absolutely!" came the enthusiastic reply. "It's one of the most important things I want to teach you! I got up at 6 am every day for probably the last 10 years of my life, and I was in bed most weeknights by 10 pm. Not only do I believe it, I *lived* it. It's one of the things that really did make a difference."

"What else is there Jake? Do you have some kind of list you need me to stick to?" I asked as a joke, but I should have known how he'd respond.

"Of course I do! They were my five foundations to making health a habit! They're easy, too: Early to bed and early to rise; stay hydrated; eat an alkaline diet; exercise every day; and relax every day."

I couldn't help but raise a cynical eyebrow.

"Wow. You were serious. I was just kidding."

"Well, Shelly, I can recommend books to read, DVDs to watch and seminars to attend and all of that is well and good for your mind. You have to also understand that your body, and how you look after it, plays as big a part. They work together. If you are in control of one, chances are you are in control of the other."

69

"It makes sense I suppose."

"I know, but...first, I want to say well done today. I'm proud of you. You did the right thing with Rob. You let him go to let him grow."

"Yes, I did. I had to. To be honest, I really wish I loved him. Out of all the guys I've gone out with, I wish I loved him more than anyone." Thinking about it was making me feel sad again.

"I understand," Jake said gently. "I felt like that with a girl I went out with once. I loved her just like you love Rob, but I wasn't in love."

"Yeah, that's it, Jake. I wasn't in love with him but I loved him, kind of like, I suppose, like I love you. I care about him."

Jake looked at me with kindness in his eyes. He understood it had been a tough thing to do.

"It's time for you both to move on, now. So let's start tonight's lesson and think about the future, ok? Early to bed, early to rise! Why? Because of two things; good sleep, and a good routine. You need to get those eight hours. Do you know what body does when you sleep?"

"Rest," I responded, suspicious of a trick question.

"Well, yes...but what I was looking for was it that recovers and repairs itself. The longer you spend in REM sleep – the longer you spend dreaming – the better you can do that. And another thing that people don't seem to realise is that we can't catch up on sleep. If you miss it, you lose the benefits. You can't make up for not sleeping on a Saturday with 12 hours on a Sunday! An hour before midnight is worth two after, as the old saying goes.

"And just as importantly, sleep turns off the thinking and worry we have while we're awake and it gives us a break from the stress of what's going on in our lives. It's an escape from our conscious worries and woes." Jake had that look he always has when he says something clever, but I quickly interrupted.

"Or, a sleep where your dead friend visits you is better than any because you wake to feel amazing no matter what you've done."

"That's true, but it's not going to last forever. I'm giving you this advice so you can start a good habit."

"I know Jake. I'm with you. Just making a joke. Did you lose your sense of humour when you died?"

He smirked.

"No, but I notice you have acquired some quick wit!"

"Well thanks, Jake. That means a lot to me!"

"Anyway, moving on. Did you know water makes up 70% of your body weight, and the human brain is 85% water? If you are not fully hydrated, it can lead to a lack of focus, concentration and even decreased intelligence."

That's a lot of water. I knew I had a bad habit of not drinking enough.

"That actually explains a lot," I told him.

"If you don't give your body enough water, it'll try to hold on to whatever it already has. Kind of like a camel going through the desert. A person can survive for up to four weeks without food, but no longer than three days without water. It's one of the best cures for most common

71

ailments; it can help with headaches, allergies, asthma, high blood pressure, diabetes, chronic fatigue and ulcers. It's the easiest way to help with weight loss. The list goes on and on! However, there isn't any money to be made in writing a prescription for water."

"I never knew that," I said.

"There was a doctor," Jake continued, "called Dr Batmanghelidj. His nickname was 'Dr Batman'. He wrote a book called *Your Body's Many Cries for Water* where he said that chronic dehydration is the root cause of most physical disease and he explained the damaging effects of dehydration."

"Cool name!" I exclaimed. "Dr Batman! So how much water should I be drinking?"

"The basic requirement is two litres per day but if you're the active type that goes up again to three."

"Oh, my God, Jake! I will be on the toilet all day if I drink that much! Does it have to be tap water? Can juice and coffee count?"

"Unfortunately not. The same goes for fizzy drinks, alcohol, tea or any caffeinated drinks for that matter. If anything, they dehydrate us more. And would you believe the *last* sign of dehydration is thirst?"

I found this a bit puzzling.

"Then how do you know you are dehydrated?"

"Well, you lack energy, you feel lethargic and you probably have sleep issues. Most headaches are caused when you're not hydrated enough. Let me ask you something...how many days would you go without having a shower?"

72

"I have a shower every day, Jake. You know that!"

"Well, there you go! You see, your insides need a wash too. Imagine when you drink water it cleans your organs and your blood, and it removes toxins from your body. You want to be like a clean waterfall, not a stagnant lake."

He'd convinced me.

"Right," I said with conviction. "As of today, I will be a waterholic."

"Good for you! And remember; the worst that can happen..."

I finished his sentence for him "...is that I feel better."

We both laughed, and he turned to me from the chair in the corner of the room. "You know," he said approvingly, "I'm seeing a real change in you already. It's great to see. It makes me so happy to be able to share it with you, and it's so good to see you being happy."

"Thank you, Jake," I said. I really meant it. I could feel the change happening too. "I want you to know I am really grateful that you have come to my rescue," I continued. "I'm feeling excited about life again, and even though it's only been a few days since you died, this has made things so much easier for me. I'm so grateful. I just wish I had listened to you more when you were alive. I mean, you really did know how to live, and I can see what an inspiration you were all along. I just feel sad that it took this to happen for me to realise it."

"Michelle Morrissey, are you actually admitting that I am totally awesome, wise, amazing, all knowing and most importantly super inspiring?"

73

I couldn't help but laugh at his cockiness.

"Yes, Jake Lawlor, I am! But only because you're dead. That's your sympathy card."

That made him laugh.

"I don't need any sympathy. I'm not suffering, depressed, worried or stressed so no need for that," he said with certainty. "But, Shelly, remember that this too will end. After our time together comes to an end, I expect you to move on and enjoy your life."

He stopped and looked up with a smile. "And on that note, class dismissed for tonight."

"What? What about the rest of the five foundations of health."

"Don't worry, Shell. There's plenty of time for them yet. Go and apply what you're learning and turn the intellectual understanding into actual understanding."

As if a jolt of electricity had passed through me, I sat upright in my bed. I looked towards the chair in the corner of the room but of course, there was no sign of Jake. The clock showed 6 am.

"Well…" I thought to myself, "it looks like I have the early to bed early to rise nailed." I giggled to myself, kicked off the covers, drank a glass of water, and decided I'd go for a walk before breakfast.

"After all," I said out loud to my empty house, "it's a lovely morning."

74

As I walked from my house to the road, I heard a voice calling. "Shelly! You decided to join the early morning club again!"

It was Troy, the postman.

"Good morning!" I greeted him. "I suppose I did. After being up at this time yesterday, I guess my body clock decided 'let's do that again today'."

"Ah I knew you would," he grinned. "Did your sister go off safely?"

"Yeah, thanks. Safe and sound! I should probably hear from her later today. Thanks for asking."

"No problem," he said happily. "I have some mail for you. Do you want me to pop it in your door?"

"Yes, please! I'm going to go for a walk so it would save me carrying them."

"No problem at all. Enjoy the walk – it's the perfect morning for it."

As I began my walk, I saw Troy walk up the pathway to my little semi-detached house. I'd lived there for nearly two years at that point, and I loved it. I bought it after Grandma Morrissey died. She had left her home to Dad, who was an only child. The family home was in Dungarvan, County Waterford. Dad grew up there. He and Mum, after much

75

consideration, sold the old cottage to a property developer. After they'd sold it, they gave each of us a gift of €10,000 to use as we pleased. I used my share as a deposit. It was probably one of the few smart things I had done in my life up to that point.

As I walked, I noticed how quiet that time of the morning really was. It was just starting to brighten up, the air was fresh and there wasn't a car to be seen. As I walked, questions popped into my head: Why hadn't I listened to Jake while he was alive? Why did Jake and his family not turn out like their father? Did Jake hate him for his temper and his violence? After walking for about an hour, I decided to return home for some breakfast and to continue reading.

When I finally arrived home I looked in the fridge. I had the feeling that Jake was probably going to advise me to make some dietary changes when I saw him later. I was by no means overweight. In fact, without sounding too cocky, I had a body most girls would die for: I was slightly curvy with a flat tummy and an average chest and bottom, but in fairness, I'd never been the most active of people. I hardly ever worked out, with the exception of the one-time Jake made me go to the gym with him. But I did meet Rob there and once I started dating him, rather than use the gym regularly I didn't bother going anymore.

I'll be the first to admit that I haven't always had the healthiest diet. I love take aways, sweets, chocolate and fizzy drinks, and I was quite partial to a few social drinks at the weekend or at home during the weekdays.

I was tired a lot and I had the reputation of being the lazy one in my family. After my conversation with Jake the night before, I began to think about my choices, and a lot of what Jake had said made sense to me. It certainly explained why I felt the way I did. I decided I needed to do a major clear-out of the fridge. As I started to throw out stuff, I realised that a lot of the contents of the fridge were out of date. Yoghurts, sauces, pre-packed meals...the only things in the fridge that were still safe to use were butter, wine and beer.

Once the fridge had been emptied and cleaned, I decided to clear out the cupboards. I became obsessed as I pulled out mouldy bread, rusty tins, and half-empty packets of pasta. I binned them all and cleaned all the presses as I went along. By the time I was finished it was nearly noon...I'd been at it for hours, but it really felt good. I took a shower and sent a text message to my Mum to ask if she'd like to meet for lunch. Her reply said *"Hey sweetheart. I was just thinking of you. Would love to meet for lunch. 1 pm hospital café?"*

I got ready and drove to the hospital to meet her. As I walked through the corridor, I was greeted by other staff members who knew me from working there. I was surprised that I didn't mind being there, even though I was off for the week and I didn't really like my job anyway. I felt different and as I walked into the canteen my mother shouted, "Shelly. Over here." She put out her arms for a hug and squeezed me tight.

Mum was a midwife at the hospital and had worked there for nearly 25 years. Everyone liked her and she had a very motherly and nurturing vibe which made her perfectly suited for her job. She looked at me with her lovely smile.

"So, my love, how is your week off going? What have you been up to?"

"Well, you'll be happy to hear that this morning I did a major clear out of my kitchen, fridge and presses. No mercy! I actually didn't notice the time go by and when I saw it was almost lunchtime and I hadn't eaten breakfast I decided to come meet you. I am starving. I haven't eaten yet."

She was both impressed and concerned, the way only a mother can be. "Well done, and in that case, we better get you some food!"

She signalled to one of the kitchen staff.

"Theresa, can we get two soups when you're ready please?"

"No problem Liz," shouted Teresa. "Anything else?"

I asked her for a tuna melt wrap and my mother pressed me for more details, asking what else I'd been doing.

"Not much really," I said, to her disappointment. "After dropping Cara off yesterday, I met Rob for a coffee, and other than that I just spent the day reading."

"You met Rob? Rob Leahy?" Mum asked, stunned.

"Yes Mum, that Rob."

"Well! What happened? Why did ye meet?"

78

"I suppose I felt it was time to deal with the whole thing, especially after Jake, and I thought we could be friends, but it seems that Rob wanted to know if there might be a chance for us in a different way."

"Of course he did. What did you say?"

Once again the memory made me feel a little down, and I started to get defensive.

"Look, Mum, I know you really like Rob and I can understand why. But I just don't love him in that way anymore, and I had to be honest. So he said if there's no hope for us, then he needs a clean break and friendship isn't on the cards. I had to let him go. You know, give him closure."

"I understand hun. I really do," she said soothingly. "And I do like Rob, but you're my daughter and I know to be truly happy in a relationship you must have that spark. You need stimulation in the head and in the bed!"

"Mum! Oh my God!" That statement shocked me but at the same time, she had a good point. She gave me a wry smile as I blushed. "That's actually quite a good way to put it, though" I admitted.

"Michelle, your father and I have an amazing marriage and I thank God every day for that man. He is all I could ask for and more, and someday you'll have that but, more importantly, you will *be* that to someone. And trust me, you won't need anyone to tell you or to give you their opinion. You'll just know."

I knew she was right, and I was sure it'd happen someday, but for now I was just going to focus on myself and my life. I told her as much, and I told her that Jake's passing had really opened my eyes and made me want to live a good life like he had.

"Good for you sweetheart," my mother said. "I know if there was ever anyone worth being inspired by, it was Jake."

Her eyes filled up at the thought of Jake. They had been very close. I leant in to comfort her.

"Ah, Mum. It's okay. You know he's in a nice place and he wouldn't want any of us to be upset."

"I know, I know," she said as she squeezed my hand. "It's just...I can remember ye all as kids. He was like a son to me. I love all the Lawlors as if they were my own. You and he were like chalk and cheese but for some reason, he always wanted to protect you. I don't know if it was because of his own childhood experiences, but he really was your guardian angel."

Mum composed herself as the food arrived at the table.

"It's fine, hun. I am just finding it a little hard and I worry for Mary after all she's been through in her life. She's like the sister I never had."

Mum was an only girl and had three older brothers. I reached across the table to hold her hand again.

"I must say, Shelly, I am very proud of how well you are dealing with this. Your father and I thought you were going to lock yourself away and take to the bed." I laughed as I remembered the first words Jake spoke to me when he first appeared.

"Yeah, I think that was a running thought in a few heads! But it didn't happen. I'm up and learning to live again. Watch this space!"

Mum laughed at me, and as we ate lunch we discussed my plans to go home and maintain my cleaning buzz. I was looking forward to getting back to it. I went straight home and tackled every wardrobe in the house, then I hoovered and polished, mopped, cleaned the bathrooms, put on a wash, cleaned the laundry room and changed the bed clothes. After dressing the bed, I glanced at the clock and was 9 pm.

"All this cleaning has me exhausted, bedtime I think." I decided to go to bed and read. Another early night, just like Jake had recommended. While reading my book, I drifted off into another deep sleep.

"Michelle Morrissey."

"Anseo!"

"You went mad with the cleaning today! I was glad to see you emptied your cupboards. That means we can fill them again, with medicine."

Jake smiled when he saw the slightly wary look on my face.

"Nature's medicine, Shell. I'm not talking Panadol and antihistamines. Healthy food is where it's at, and it's medicine you can take every day! We're going to achieve balance!"

I sat up and listened attentively.

"Homoeostasis is the word of the day. It's the sweet spot between acidity and alkalinity. When our acid/alkaline balance is disturbed, it is a precursor to all sorts of sensitivities and diseases."

81

This all seemed to be getting very scientific.

"Right...homoeostasis. Cool. So...how do we do that?"

"Well, your blood's pH level should be slightly alkaline. Your blood can become too acidic because of an acidic diet, or emotional stress, dehydration and so on. When that happens the body will try to compensate by using alkaline minerals...but if your diet doesn't have enough minerals to compensate, you get a build-up of acid and it starts to affect your whole system."

"Jesus Jake, that sounds kind of scary." I was worried.

"It is! But we can fix it and prevent it with a well-balanced diet; full of fresh, live foods. Your diet ought to be 75%-80% alkaline foods."

"How am I supposed to know which foods to eat?!"

Jake was obviously revelling in my consternation and found time for a dramatic pause before he answered me.

"It's easy! Go green! Eat as many vegetables, fruit and salads as possible. Choose white meat and seafood instead of red meat. Go for yeast-free bread, wild rice and potatoes. Choose to drink coconut or almond milk instead of cow's milk. Use coconut oil or cold pressed olive oil instead of saturated fats or butter."

I was beginning to think this list of instructions would be too much to remember, but Jake was on a roll.

"If you're going to sit down and watch TV, go for a 30-minute walk beforehand for balance. It's also very important to reduce stress as much as possible. Try meditation or yoga, or some other relaxing method to restore inner peace!"

I think my eyes must have started to glaze over because Jake put his head to one side and raised his eyebrows. It was his 'are you paying attention?' face. I raised mine in return...it was my 'yes, just keep going' face.

"You may not know it, but back-lit screens can throw your chemistry out too. Blue light forces your brain to make substances it can't use up quickly at night. I know you love your laptop and your phone, but try to cut them out late at night. Then, there's the usual stuff we all know about, like not smoking, not drinking alcohol and not taking medication and painkillers unless really necessary."

"There's a lot to take in there Jake, I can't help but feel a little overwhelmed."

"Okay, I know it's a lot!" he laughed. "Keep it simple: Eat fresh! Your fridge should be fuller than your freezer. Aim for balance. Does that make sense?"

"Yeah it all makes sense but it sounds like a lot of work. This is all easy for you to say, you don't have to worry about it anymore! What else have you got for me?"

"Keep a food diary for a month and just record what you are eating and how you feel. You'll start to see a pattern associated with certain foods."

"Now *that's* a good idea!" I said. Finally, something that seemed obvious!

Jake laughed at my obvious relief. "You know I'm not really telling you anything you don't already know! It's more like I'm highlighting things. But we have to move on to a subject you know absolutely nothing about now."

I braced myself.

"It's a very strange and very difficult concept for you: exercise."

"Ha ha! Very funny Jake."

"Come on," he chuckled, "it's no secret that you might just be the laziest person in Castletown!"

I burst into a fit of laughter.

"I knew you would do this Jake! Okay, I was lazy but I will make an effort I swear. Besides wasn't I out walking this morning at 6.30am, for goodness sake?"

"True Shell and I think that's a super start, but you will have to make it as much a habit as going to work or brushing your teeth okay?"

"I will, I swear. The change is on, my friend."

"It'll be a change for the better! Exercise is good for your heart and bones, slows down ageing, helps prevent disease, improves your sex life, lowers blood pressure, improves brain function and affects energy levels and sleep. Exercising even creates endorphins which are the happy hormones, so it improves your mood!"

"Sold, Jake. I get it! Make it a habit just like you did, blah blah blah! What got you into sports in the first place Jake? I don't remember you ever not doing sports?"

"It was just natural to me. Remember how I was soccer-mad in primary school, like every other boy? I only ended up playing rugby when I went to secondary. I loved moving and pushing myself and

84

competing...but it wasn't just for the physical benefits, ever. It was more the mental side of it. I suppose it got me to be a mental athlete as well as a physical one, so to speak. I remember we were around 15 when Martin, Brian and I started to go Thai Boxing every Tuesday evening."

I remembered it well. We all thought Jake was on his way to becoming a ninja warrior. I was getting piano lessons from his brother Michael at the time, and Mike would drop him to the club on his way to teach me.

"We were all playing on the under-16 football team and the Thai Boxing was an extra training session but not a priority to any of us," Jake continued, taking a break from advising me to reminisce instead. "I remember one evening, all the lads pulled out of going for whatever reasons and I decided to go anyway. I'll never forget it. I had no partner, so I was paired up with the coach for a few rounds and I ended up getting sick and everything. Fit as I thought I was, it pushed me to a new place and, as strange as it might sound, it felt really good. It was just me. No team, just me."

I remembered this part of his life well. He ended up going every week, and then twice a week, and then on Saturday morning too when soccer season was over. He was definitely bitten by the bug.

"It gave me a different release to any other sport I had done," Jake explained. "I wasn't as angry, even with all that was happening at home. It even improved my performance in other sports. That's when I started lifting weights and it progressed from there. Weight training really improves your focus. You only have to look at Arnold Schwarzenegger to know that's true!" There's a man who decides what he wants and gets it."

"Interesting stuff Jake, but I don't really want to be like Arnie!"

"Why not? He's inspirational! He was the world's most famous bodybuilder, and he said he wanted to be in movies. People laughed at him. What did he do? He became a huge movie star! Then he decided he wanted to be in politics. People laughed. What did he do? He became the Governor of California! Sounds pretty inspirational to me!"

"Ok...but could I do something like that without all the muscles?"

"Well," he answered, looking at my biceps, "maybe not as *much* muscle! But some muscle is good! Not enough people know this, but muscle actually burns fat. So the more muscle you have, the less fat you have and the leaner and more toned you become."

I had to grin. This was definitely the sports-mad, passionate Jake I'd known and loved.

"You're like my own personal nutritionist and trainer," I laughed.

"Shelly, there are plenty of nutritionists and personal trainers out there. Besides you are better off to pay someone and, maybe for you, it would be better if you don't know them."

"Why?"

"Well, you never listened to me until I died. So, from experience, maybe a stranger would be more suitable!"

"Good point."

"Start as you mean to go on, Shell. Now, we're going to have to say goodbye again but you have lots to do to keep you busy, and then when we meet again you can look forward to learning about how to relax."

"Didn't you just tell me I need the opposite?!"

He didn't answer, and I realised I was fully awake.

I turned over in bed and glanced at the clock. Shock horror, it was 6 am again, on another fresh morning. The sun shone in my window, and I decided I'd go for a walk, seeing as I was awake. I'd need to get some food, seeing as I'd thrown nearly everything out the day before, and I had an overwhelming urge to speak to someone about a health and fitness plan.

As I made my way downstairs I felt a little cramp in my stomach. It was back, worse the second time, as I got to the bottom of the stairs. I tried to ignore it, but within a few minutes, I had to run to the bathroom to get sick. I spent most of the morning running to the toilet, on the toilet, or over the toilet. I threw myself across the couch. What a perfect time to be hit with some sort of mystery bug. I decided to text the only person I knew who would know what to do.

'*Hey Mum. Can you buzz me when you are free, please? Xxx*'

I lay there sipping water until the phone rang.

"Hey Mum. Thanks for calling me."

"No problem love. Everything okay?"

"Not really. I think I have a bug."

"Oh no sweetheart! What are your symptoms?"

"Well, I woke up feeling fine. Then, out of nowhere, I got cramps. By the time I made it downstairs, I was bent over in pain. I spent the morning in the bathroom."

"Poor doll! Are you vomiting or do you have diarrhoea?"

"Both! I am just sipping water at the moment."

"Right, firstly no water."

"No water? But won't I get dehydrated? I can't keep anything down or in!"

"I know sweetheart, but it sounds like a gastric bug and water is only going to go right through you too. I will pop over on my lunch and bring you a magic cure; some Imodium for the diarrhoea and electrolytes to keep you hydrated, okay?" I glanced at the clock; it was 11.15am.

"Thanks, Mum, what time are you on lunch?"

"1 pm sweetheart, will you be okay till then?"

"Yeah, I'll survive. Thanks, Mum. See you then."

"Look, sweetie, just stay near the toilet and relax till I get there okay."

"Okay Mum, bye."

I turned on the TV and just lay there. I could feel sweat on my skin as I doubled over with more cramps. I must have spent the following two hours between the toilet and the couch. As I flushed for what seemed like the millionth time, I heard my mother's voice.

"How's the patient?"

I walked out of the bathroom like a zombie.

"Hey Mum. Not so good, to be honest."

89

"Jesus, Shell, you look terrible!"

I winced.

"Thanks, Mum. That makes me feel much better."

"Poor baby, you just lie on that couch and I will fix you right up."

"Thanks for coming over on your lunch Mum."

"No problem sweetheart, I couldn't have one of my babies sick now, could I? Here drink this." She handed me a can of Coca-Cola.

"Drink that straight back now Shelly. That will sort you right out."

"What? Really? Coke?"

"Yes, really, Coke! By the looks of it, you have the tummy bug that's rampant in the hospital at the moment. This will have you right as rain in no time."

"Whatever you say, Mum. I'll try anything."

I drank the can of coke and sat back on the couch. Mum sat next to me.

"What if it doesn't work Mum? What else can I do? I mean I will have to drink something."

"I brought you some electrolytes to replace lost fluids and minerals, and some Imodium in case you still have diarrhoea later, okay?"

"Yeah. Thanks, Mum."

My mother put her arms around me and guided me down to lie across her lap. She rubbed my hair and asked, "Shell, have I told you about the lovely old couple who are in the hospital at the moment?"

"No Mum. You haven't."

"Well we have a lady named Nuala who has Alzheimer's and she's in Ward B on the second floor. And her husband, Teddy, has cancer and he's at the other side of the hospital. I swear Shell, it's like a movie. Almost every day, as sick as he is, he makes the journey over to Ward B to visit her. And every day she tells him to go away, "If my husband sees you, he will get very cross," she tells him. It's just so sad to watch. I swear half the nurses are in tears by the time the visit is over. And that poor man makes his way back to his ward and waits 'till the next day to try again, hoping she will recognise him."

"Is this supposed to make me feel better Mum?"

Mum laughed, "Not really. Just wanted to distract you for a bit. How are you feeling now?"

"I'm not sure yet. I haven't had a cramp anyway, Oh, excuse me," I belched. Mum frowned and laughed.

"That's the Coke working, I'd say! You shouldn't have any more diarrhoea or vomiting. After an hour or so, drink some coconut water to replace any lost fluids, and more this evening before bed too. I'd better head back to the hospital, will you be okay?"

"Yeah, I'm good now Mum. I will probably head to bed later. I feel wrecked from being sick."

"Do that sweetheart. Go to bed and get a good night's sleep and you will wake right as rain. It's only a 24-hour bug so don't eat or drink any water, just sleep it off."

"Thanks, Mum."

"If you need anything, let me know."

"I will Mum. Thanks again."

After Mum left I watched TV for a while. As I flicked through the channels looking for something good to watch, I felt a wave of exhaustion come over me, so I decided to just go to bed. I thought of Jake and decided that if I went to bed and slept, I'd wake up feeling better. Why didn't I think of it sooner? I slowly made my way upstairs and turned on the heating. It wasn't even four o'clock but I was completely exhausted. I got under the covers, turned over in the bed and started to rub my belly.

"Are you okay?" came a familiar voice.

"Hey Jake! Well, I seem to be now. Thanks."

"Yeah, bugs suck! Especially when it comes out both ends."

I scowled at him. The mental image was the last thing I needed.

"The Coke is working wonders, though, right?" He was right, it really did seem to be making a difference for the better. I told him so.

"Mum used to say it went right through you and ripped the bug right up and out of the body. It always worked when we were kids anyway!" he proclaimed.

"I think it did the trick for me anyway Jake. I felt better when I went to bed. I was just tired from the whole thing."

"Yeah, it can knock you for six."

"Distract me!" I ordered him "Continue the lessons!"

Of course, he obliged.

"I suppose this is as good a time as to appreciate your health and to learn to change the way you look at illness," he said, sounding serious again.

"Okay Jake, I get the 'appreciate the health' thing. But what do you mean by 'learn to change the way you look at illness?'"

"Illness is usually your body telling you something. It's a sign that there is stress or pressure where there shouldn't be. Issues in your tissues, so to speak."

"Ha ha! Issues in your tissues! I like it!"

"Shelly do you remember I mentioned Dr Batmanghelidj."

"Yeah, sure. Dr Batman!"

"That's him! He was convinced that most of the time when people feel sick, all they need is water. Simple. It reminds me of Occam's razor: *All things being equal, the simplest solution tends to be the best one.*"

"I think I heard Lisa Simpson say that once..." I told him.

"Yeah, you probably did."

"So why are you telling me about Occam's Razor?"

"Because the quickest, simplest solution to a problem is usually the right one, and it works far better for all involved as opposed to over-analysing and overthinking. Dr Batman thought it was as simple as water. Today for you, it was Coke. Sometimes we ignore the most obvious solutions while we look for some profound meaning or complicated explanation as to why things aren't going our way."

93

"I can see that," I replied, "but sometimes it's not that simple. I mean, when people have cancer or other life-threatening diseases, water or Coke aren't going to do much good. I think it's a little bit more complicated than that!"

"Do you think complicating it is the solution?" he countered.

"Well…" I said, "what do you suggest?"

"Prevention," he stated with certainty. "People need to learn to focus on what they want rather than what they don't want. If you want health, focus on health. If you want money, focus on money. If you want love, focus on love. If you want joy, fun and laughter, focus on them!"

"Sounds simple, Jake, but if that was the case everyone would be doing it."

"Really? Last time I checked, most people tend to focus on what they don't want."

After my horrible day, I was feeling a little more argumentative than usual. "That's a bit extreme," I said bluntly. "Nobody wants to be sick. I sure didn't want to be sick today."

"I'm not saying that Shell," Jake said patiently. "What I am saying, is that when people do get sick, that's what occupies their minds. Take my buddy Mike as an example. You remember Mike?"

I did. Mike had very bad arthritis and was hardly able to walk without his walking stick. He'd been like that as long as I'd known him: if he walked 50 yards he would have to sit down for a rest as the pain in his legs was too unbearable.

"Have you seen him lately? I mean in the last year or so?"

94

"He was at your funeral."

"Did you notice anything different?"

As a matter of fact, I had. At the funeral, Mike had seemed a lot more mobile than I remembered, and I mentioned that to Jake.

"Exactly!" he exclaimed. "Mike decided he'd had enough pain and suffering. He made the relevant changes to his lifestyle. He took action and focused on being well. He focused on walking around easily. He focused on health."

"Are you saying he got rid of his arthritis?"

"If you were to meet Mike now and ask him how his arthritis was, he would tell you, 'It's not my arthritis.' He has it under control – he doesn't let it control him."

"Jake, do you really believe that people can cure themselves of illness?"

"Think of all those times in your life, just like today, when you got sick, or times when you cut yourself or broke a bone. Did you die?"

"Obviously not."

"Exactly, because your body healed itself in the best way it knew how and I am guessing it did it in the quickest and simplest way too."

"I suppose you're right."

"Shelly, it doesn't matter who's right or wrong really. What matters is what works, and your body works for you. When you get a cut, it heals. When you get sick, your immune system makes you better. I'm saying, try not to worry or stress out and trust your body to do what it

95

needs to do. I'm saying take the necessary steps to keep yourself out of pain so you can focus on wellness.

"We tend to underestimate our own abilities – especially our ability to heal. We are all natural born healers, but the best solution is to concentrate on staying well in the first place. In ancient China, the emperor's doctor was paid to keep the emperor healthy and well; if the Emperor fell ill, the doctor was not paid."

"If that happened nowadays, doctors would be broke," I mused.

"Maybe. Or maybe more people would be healthy rather than sick. Maybe a change of attitude wouldn't hurt."

I admitted that I hadn't thought of that. It's funny where we place our values. We pay for health care for when we get sick but most of us don't put the same value on our health.

"It should be called sick care, not health care," I said.

"Good point!" Jake responded. "It seems so strange but that's us. Strange humans."

I could sense that our time was nearly up, and I wasn't surprised when Jake said he had to go.

"Stay healthy and remember, you are responsible for your health: focus on it."

"I will, Jake, thanks."

Then, suddenly, I was awake, and he was gone.

As I lay in bed for a while daydreaming, I was very grateful to be well again. Jake's encouragement had worked, and I felt like today was an action day. I had lots to do and lots to plan. I was going to take the first steps towards a new, healthy lifestyle.

As well as my mission to find a nutritionist and a personal trainer, I knew I'd also have to prepare for 'Trick Or Treaters' later that night, as it was Hallowe'en. I put on my coat to go out and noticed that it seemed a little more snug than usual. "Good thing I'm going to get a nutritionist," I thought to myself. As I walked out the door, Troy was on his way up the path.

"Good morning, Troy. Beautiful morning isn't it?"

"That it is, Michelle. That it is. I knew it wouldn't take long until you got into starting your days early. It's great, don't you think?"

"I suppose it's got its advantages," I agreed. "It's peaceful."

He handed me a sheaf of letters and bills, and I thanked him before wishing him well. He turned around and set out on his way. As we parted company, I remembered what Jake said just before I had woke that morning: "Say hi to Troy for me."

I shouted after him before all of a sudden realising what I was about to say and how crazy it would sound.

97

Troy turned around and looked back at me. I had to think fast.

"Oh...uh...I was just wondering how is your little girl, Amelie?" Not the worst cover-up in the world...it seemed to do the trick.

"Oh, she's just magic!" beamed the proud father. "Thanks for asking."

"No problem, have a great day."

"You too."

I popped back into my house, placed the letters on the table inside the hall door and laughed to myself. That could have been a disaster. I closed the front door, set out on my walk and started to imagine the shape I wanted to achieve. I thought about how much better I was going to feel and I started to get excited about the idea of changing habits and taking up a hobby. After walking for about an hour, I stopped at the shop on my way back home. I got there just as they opened at 7.30, and as I approached the door I heard someone calling me, "Shelly Morrissey. What, in the name of God, are you doing up at this time of the morning?" It was my younger sister Eve.

"Hiya Evie!" I said with a smile "I was out walking and I needed to get something for my breakfast, so here I am."

"A walk? You? God, what time did you get up at?"

"Six."

"What? Seriously?! But you're still off work, aren't you?"

I found her incredulity quite entertaining. It was nice to catch her off guard and I had to grin as I answered her.

98

"Yes, but I got up early and went for a walk. I plan on doing it regularly from now on. Is it really that shocking?"

"Sorry Shell. It's just not like you."

"I know Eve, but people change."

I could tell she was impressed, but of course, she was doing her best to hide it. She seized the moment and asked me to join her for breakfast at the Coffee Dock before she headed to college. "Sister Time," she called it. We walked across the road to the Coffee Dock and sat by the window in our customary spot. The girl behind the counter, Jen, knew us both. Eve, always hungry, ordered Eggs Benedict and coffee the moment we sat down, and I went for Eggs Florentine with some brown bread.

Eve stared at me with renewed surprise.

"What?" I couldn't help but ask as she sat there with her mouth practically gaping open.

"Eggs Florentine? What about the usual full Irish? Next, you're going to be telling me you're going on a diet and joining a gym!"

"Actually I am looking for a good gym or personal trainer. Do you know of any good ones?"

Eve blinked with exaggerated slowness and shook her head from side to side.

"Ok. Seriously. Who are you, and what have you done with my sister?"

"Smart-ass!" I laughed. "I just want to make a few changes. Big deal. Jake's death has made me look at things differently, and I want to improve my life. I want to be better. Aren't you the one always preaching about making positive changes?" She looked at me a little closer, and then I wasn't just getting coffee with my baby sister; I was having breakfast with a psychology student.

"I understand Jake's passing is hard on you, and I'm glad to hear you want to improve your life like Jake did, but…" she was clearly making an effort to be diplomatic; "it just sounds like you're turning into Jake overnight. It's just very quick."

I had to admit that she was right, but I wasn't going to just let her off the hook about her own efforts to change me: "you're the one who's always telling me that procrastination is the mother of all evils, Eve. So, are you going to help me or not?"

She grabbed her bag and pulled out a business card and a pen, scribbled a name on it and handed it to me. I flipped it over and read it.

"'The Gym'. Where's that?"

"These guys are great for fast results and proper monitoring," said Eve. "It's along the Quays. It's a personal training studio, which means you get a trainer and a nutritionist. If you really are serious, then this is the best place for you. I did a programme there a few years ago, remember?"

"Oh yeah! You raved about the place, but you said it was really strict."

"Well, yeah Shell, but only if you're not used to eating clean. Besides, it's professional and you will feel and see a difference, and you'll get the motivation you need to get you into the training side of things. Talk to Ivan. He's the manager. I know him from the college and he's the reason I went there in the first place. I've sent a load of people his way since, as well, so he'll look after you well."

After breakfast, we went our separate ways, Eve to college and me to pick up my bits and pieces at the shop before going home. When I arrived back it was nearly 9 am. I decided to call The Gym.

"Hello. May I speak to Ivan, please?"

"This is Ivan speaking."

"Hi, Ivan. My name is Michelle Morrissey. My sister, Eve, told me to ask for you. I want to enquire about joining The Gym."

"Great, Michelle. I am very happy to help Eve's sister. If you are around today, pop over and see the place and I can go through everything with you in person."

We chatted for a while and finally agreed to meet at The Gym at 4 pm. By the time I hung up the phone, I was very impressed and very excited about going. I put my shopping away and went upstairs to fish out my training gear. It was nowhere to be found, so I delved a little deeper.

As I rummaged through my wardrobe, I found a nun's habit. It was an old fancy dress costume. A sly thought crept into my head: Why not make use of the costume, seeing as it was Hallowe'en? I could wear it for the trick-or-treaters. It wasn't exactly gym appropriate, however, so I knew I'd have to make another trip to the shops for some sweatpants and a light top.

Apart from that unplanned excursion, I spent the rest of the day organising decorations and treats for Halloween. I had invited my friends Claire and Fran over for dinner and drinks and convinced them to dress up for Halloween. I was in the mood for some fun.

At 4 pm, I arrived at The Gym to meet Ivan. As I walked into the reception area, I was greeted by a young girl behind the desk. "Good afternoon, welcome to 'The Gym'. My name is Diane. How can I help you?"

"Hi, Diane. My name is Michelle Morrissey. I have an appointment with Ivan."

"Are you Eve's sister?" she asked enthusiastically. "It's great to meet you!" She walked around the desk and shook my hand. Ivan is just finishing a consultation. He won't be long."

I sat down and watched as a few people walked in. Diane greeted them all with a smile and guided them into the gym area for their training session. I read a health magazine and took it all in. A trainer walked towards me.

"Hello," he greeted me. "Nice day, isn't it?"

"Yes, it is."

"Are you joining us?" he asked before Diane interrupted.

"Mark, this is Eve's sister."

"No way!" he exclaimed. "It's so nice to meet you!" He extended his arm to shake my hand and he and Diane joked that they'd have to make sure I am well looked after. Eve must have made quite an impression while she was working out there. I was already very impressed, and just at that moment a tall, incredibly handsome man arrived and made a bee-line for me.

"Michelle, sorry to keep you waiting. I am Ivan."

He reached out his hand to shake mine and I could barely string a sentence together. He was a vision.

"Follow me this way," he told me. I tottered after him, still dumbstruck.

Ivan directed me to his office, and we went through the usual small talk. He was not only ridiculously attractive but also very pleasant and friendly. It was almost too good to be true. Finally, we got down to the matter at hand.

"So, Michelle. Tell me what it is you're looking for, and let's see what I can do for you."

I paused for a second and a thought that had absolutely nothing to do with what he was asking me passed through my mind. Aware that I was probably staring at him, I composed myself and responded.

"Well, Ivan...uh...I want to improve my health and fitness and I suppose I wouldn't mind losing a few kilos along the way."

I smiled, slightly embarrassed by what I had just said to this fine specimen in front of me.

"Well, Michelle..."

"Shelly. It's Shelly. My friends...I mean...call me Shelly. Please."

I appeared to have entered the babbling stage. I blushed. He smiled.

"Okay, Shelly. The fitness and health; no problem. As for the weight, you don't need to lose any."

Music to my ears. I was acutely aware of the idiotic grin which spread across my face.

"It's more about tightening up, if anything," he continued. "When people come here to train, they're educated on good nutrition for health and fuelling the body for performance. We give them all the tools, but when they succeed at achieving their goals, it's their own personal success. Of course, if they don't take our advice and guidance and they fail, then that's their own failure too, but that's rare. While you're training here, we'll make sure you have everything you need to get the results you desire; the best nutritional food plans, top quality training, inspiration and a positive mental climate. How does that sound?"

"It sounds great!" I said, but what I think I really meant was "you're great!"

Ivan treated me to a huge grin. "Okay then! So, before I bring you into the gym and get one of the trainers to explain the programme to you, when do you want to start?"

"I suppose tomorrow if I can?"

"Great! I can do your consultation today if you like, and you can train first thing in the morning. How does that sound?"

"Perfect."

I'd hoped I'd get to spend more time with Ivan, but he had a lot to do so another staff member guided me through the training programme and showed me the weights and machines. The buzz in the gym was electric. After the induction, I was given a food plan, weighed, measured and passed back to Diane for paperwork. She set up my appointments, took payment and showed me the changing room. As I drove home, I couldn't stop thinking about the gym and the atmosphere there. And Ivan. Lovely, lovely Ivan.

When I got back I prepared dinner; my 'last supper' before I went on my new eating plan. The girls arrived in their fancy dress. I had my nun outfit on, Claire was a ninja and Fran was a genie. We ate, drank wine and greeted the neighbourhood children as they went trick or treating around the estate. The girls filled me in on all the gossip and I told them all about the gym, with passing mention of Ivan and his remarkable hotness. After all the gossiping was over, the girls left, I cleaned up and headed for bed. I had to be at the gym at 7 am in the morning and I could hardly wait to get to sleep.

I hopped into bed and I drifted off in no time, my mind full of thoughts of a tall, handsome gym owner.

"Do you have a soft spot already for your new fitness coach?"

I sat upright in my bed, eager to chat about my action-packed day.

"I wouldn't put it like that, Jake! I would say I just have an appreciation for beautiful things and he is very beautiful."

"Fair enough. I won't argue with you."

Jake paced back and forth across the room and then sat in the chair in the corner, as he usually did.

"I have an important question for you." I was all ears. "Do you think you know how to relax?"

I took a moment to here to think.

"Well, I always presumed that when I was doing nothing in particular, maybe, just chilling on the couch watching TV and I wasn't working, then I was relaxing. I'm guessing you're going to tell me I'm not, though." Jake looked like he was sizing up my interpretation and paused uncharacteristically before he replied.

"Well, you're not wrong! To most of the world, sitting on the sofa and watching television *is* relaxing, and in comparison to their jobs and work it probably feels that way. But you're right; that isn't what I'm referring to. When I say relaxation or meditation, I mean preparing and clearing the mind for good experiences. Do you know what to do to accomplish that?"

"No, clearly I don't!"

"Nothing Shell, sweet, nothing."

"Okay Jake, I am not sure what you mean."

"Well, you know the way that most people think that meditation is when you just stop thinking?" I nodded. "And relaxation is clearing the mind?" I nodded again. "It's not. Your mind is like your wardrobe and there are some clothes in there that you have for years, some are too small, some are too big, some you have never worn, some you have

106

worn out, some are in fashion and some have never been and never will be in fashion.

"But, every now and again, you go to the wardrobe and do a spring clean. You get rid of some of the old stuff that you never used and wonder why you had it, and you buy some new clothes to suit your current lifestyle. It's like today when you bought new training gear. It's not about throwing out everything. You just get rid of what doesn't suit you anymore and you focus on the clothes that do.

"So if you want to relax, don't throw out all your thoughts. Observe them. Focus on the ones that make you feel good. Focus on the ones you want in your life. When you become the observer, there is nothing to do; it's effortless. You can concentrate on the good thoughts and grow them, and examine the not-so-good thoughts and let them go. Are you with me?"

"Yeah, kind of," I answered. It all seemed to make sense. "Let my thoughts happen, and then...well, think about my thoughts? Then decide which ones to keep thinking?"

"Yeah, that's it, Shell! Very good. I actually remember when I started doing relaxation. I was around 26 years old and I was dating Karen."

I remembered Karen. She was a total hippy chick. A really nice girl.

"She was great. She took me to a few relaxation classes and meditation classes. But, I really liked this one particular class. The woman doing the class, Esther, was really kind and sweet and when she spoke everything she said made sense. One time she said 'Not relaxing is like trying to get from Cork to Dublin, and you can't find your car keys so you decide to walk.' It's choosing to take the hard way."

"Was that the Monday night class you used to go to?"

"Yeah. Every Monday night for nearly seven years."

"And was Karen still there all that time too?"

"No, she moved to Germany shortly after we broke up. Anyway, there is a quote from Ernest Hemingway that I really like: '*If something is wrong, then fix it if you can, but train yourself not to worry: Worry never fixes anything.*'"

That one appealed to me, and I told Jake so.

"Relaxation ought to be about releasing our worries and igniting our desires," he said. "I think some Monday you should just take a visit to the class with Esther. I think you'll really get something out of it, especially now."

"Ok, sure! I'll give it a go. Nothing ventured, nothing gained. But! Speaking of venturing and gaining...what do you think of my action today? The Gym; did you know about this place? It's really different and I feel really excited about starting my programme."

"I know everything, Shelly. I thought we discussed this,"

I giggled.

"I trained there during soccer season last year. It's awesome. Even you will love it," Jake joked.

"I'm so excited about it!" I enthused. "I never imagined that I'd be excited about going to a gym!"

"You see?" he asked with a grin. "You're starting to become aware of the possibilities. And you're putting out a far nicer vibe and energy so other people's kindness and positivity are what you get in return!"

"Yeah, that's so true. I am really starting to feel the difference. But...what happens when you're gone, Jake? How will I feel then? How will I feel in the mornings, when I don't have a Jake sleep?"

Jake looked at me with an expression of deep love and kindness. It was the same look he always gave me when I was in danger of freaking out or of losing faith in myself.

"Shelly, that is entirely up to you. But I know you, and I'm sure you'll be just as ready and up for it as you are now. I promise; when we're finished with our time together, you will be in a far better place mentally and physically. This will all be second nature to you. And more than anything, I know you'll be fine."

"Do you really think so?" I asked in a small voice.

"Yes Shelly, I know so." Jake smiled at me and I instantly felt better.

"Okay, then," he said gently. "It's nearly time for your first training session. I can't wait to hear all about it later. Good luck, Shell."

*Chapter 10 - Sleep 10*

*Friday 1ˢᵗ November*

I woke up and lay there basking for a few minutes, paying attention to my thoughts as they zipped around my head, one after another, after another. There didn't seem to be any gaps. After a while, I got out of bed and got ready for the gym. It was 6.15am. I decided that this would be the time I would go to the gym most mornings.

While brushing my teeth I started to hum *Galileo* again. It had been in my head now for a fortnight! I made a mental note to ask Jake if he knew why. When I was ready for the gym, I made my way to the car, bumping into Troy on the way.

"Hello Shelly!" came the cheery greeting. "Another beautiful morning, isn't it?"

"It sure is Troy! Smashing!"

"No post today, pet."

"No news is good news!" I grinned. "It's a relief, actually: I'm on my way to The Gym and it's my first session so it might be a hard morning. Bills would have been an unwelcome distraction!"

"Not to worry," he said kindly. "What doesn't kill us makes us stronger, as they say!"

I promised him I'd bear that in mind as I sat into my car and drove the back roads to The Gym. I made sure to give myself a little extra

110

time that morning to freshen up, just in case a certain someone was working early. As I approach the car park, I started to feel butterflies. "Oh my God Michelle Morrissey," I scolded my reflection in the rear-view mirror: "Get a grip of yourself!" I took a moment to make sure I was settled, got out of the car and headed up to The Gym. It was a really fresh morning and felt just like autumn should; it was dry and sunny and everything looked orange. I was greeted by a very cheery Diane.

"Good morning, Shelly! All set for day one?"

"I sure am!" I shot back. "I was born ready!"

She laughed.

"Excellent! Well, this morning you will have the pleasure of being trained by the lovely Nicky. She is tough but very sweet."

I couldn't help but feel a little disappointed. I really wanted to see Ivan. But I told myself that at least I'd see him again soon, and besides, it was probably for the best that he didn't see me all sweaty and red faced! As I drifted off into my thoughts, I was quickly brought back into the moment when I heard someone calling my name.

"Michelle?"

I looked up to see a beautiful young woman, with dark hair, sallow skin, sparkly blue eyes and a warm smile.

"Hello, Michelle. I'm Nicky and I'll be your trainer today."

I couldn't help but feel like I knew this girl, she was very familiar.

"Hi Nicky," I said. "Have we met before?"

111

"Yes, I know you! And by the end of the workout you'll remember me too," she said cryptically. "I know your sister Eve very well; she's some girl to train."

"Oh God, Nicky! I am the odd one out in the family. Both my sisters are like Superwoman compared to me!"

"Not for long, Michelle!" she stated confidently. "Not when you are done here."

"Well, I have literally done nothing in about two and a half years except walk to and from my car."

Nicky laughed at me but I am sure she was thinking, 'Lazy Bitch!' I looked at her and told her earnestly that I wasn't kidding, and she looked right back at me with what suddenly seemed to be the most genuine, caring eyes I had ever seen.

"I understand, don't worry. I promise I am going to take care of you today: I'll show you each exercise so you can see it, I'll talk you through them just because I like to talk, and then I'll explain where you are going to feel each exercise so you'll know what muscles you're working. No pressure, no pain, just an introduction to weight lifting. Okay? The worst that can happen at the end of the session is you feel better!"

Nicky smiled at me for a while with a knowing look on her face. It was like she was waiting for a reaction. Then, all of a sudden, she got one. I almost jumped out of my skin.

"Oh, Nicky! I am so sorry. It's been years since I've seen you. God, I feel so silly."

Her smile broadened into a grin.

"Wow! That line is all it took, Michelle. Well done! I thought it would be at least the end of the session before you remembered."

Nicky was an old flame of Jake's. They met while travelling years ago and stayed together for a few months. After Jake returned home, Nicky kept travelling and only came back the odd Christmas. Jake and she had stayed friends. He'd always been good at staying on good terms with his exes.

"How long have you been back?"

"Oh, I've worked here on and off for about five years. I go travelling every now and then for a few months and I am blessed that Ivan takes me back each time. We're cousins."

"Oh! Ivan is your cousin. I see. That's very handy."

"Yeah it really is, he's great. So, how are you getting on at the moment? I wanted to come talk to you after the funeral but I didn't think you would remember me and you were so bombarded by people."

"You were at the funeral?"

"Yes, I was. I think the whole of Cork was at that funeral, Michelle"

"Oh, call me Shelly, please."

"Okay, Shelly. Enough chit-chat! We'd better get you training, or it'll be lunch time!"

We went through the training induction and afterwards, Nicky walked me back to reception. I actually felt fine. I mean, I felt like I worked my muscles but I didn't feel wrecked. It wasn't what I'd expected. I hit the showers and changed to go in town for a little shopping. As I walked back into reception, Ivan and Mark were standing behind the desk.

"How was day one?" asked Ivan.

"Hey guys," I replied, as cool as possible. "Yeah good. Trained the legs! In fact, I could probably do it again."

They both looked at me a little incredulously. I resisted an urge to giggle, play with my hair and bat my eyelashes at Ivan, but somehow I managed to retain my composure.

"I'm kidding. It was great, thanks. I am sure I'll feel them tomorrow!"

"Yeah, you probably will," Mark said with a smile.

"Don't mind him, Shelly," said Ivan. "What's your plan for the day now? Off to work?"

"No, I'm off shopping, I'm on holidays till next Monday, so I am going to enjoy the last few days."

"Good for you!" Ivan replied. "Will I see you tomorrow morning?"

I wanted to shout "YES, PLEASE!" but I forced myself to be more refined: "I suppose you will if you're here at 9 am."

"I'll be here," he promised with a smile as I made my way to the door.

I wanted some new clothes and, seeing as it was my dad's birthday, I had to pick up a birthday present. I shopped until lunchtime, then met the girls from the band for coffee and a catch-up. We mostly talked about the gym and, inevitably, lovely, lovely Ivan. By the time we stopped nattering it was 4 pm. I hadn't even noticed.

"Wow, girls!" I said once I realised. "I'd better get going! I have my Dad's birthday dinner. I'll be in touch next week to check the schedule, okay?"

"Okay, Shell. Say Happy Birthday to Gary!"

"Yeah, tell your dad to have a fabulous birthday."

Traffic wasn't too heavy so I popped home for a quick costume change and to wrap Dad's present. Then, out the door again to my parents' house. Morrissey family birthday dinners are a tradition. For every birthday in the family, we get together for dinner and birthday boy or girl gets to pick whatever cake they want. After dinner, I attempted to get up to go to the bathroom but my legs didn't seem to be working as they normally would. They were starting to feel really sore.

"Oh my God, my legs are broken!" I lamented. "I didn't expect to be this sore after my first session! Wow!" I limped back over to sit at the kitchen table, ignoring the laughter from the family.

Mum dimmed the lights and brought out the birthday cake and we all sang *Happy Birthday* to my father. We gathered around and gave him a big hug, and then we started to give him our gifts, one after the other. After the presents were open and my slice of cake was gone, I decided it was time to make my way home. I was so sore and so exhausted, I felt like I was sure to go into a coma when I got there.

115

I started to get up from the table and I couldn't help but leave out a little whimper from the pain in my muscles. Eve gave a knowing laugh.

"Don't worry Shelly, it will get easier!" she promised. "Besides, tomorrow you train your arms so you won't do your legs again until next week."

"Thanks," I said. "Will I give you a shout in the morning after the gym to see if you want to join me for breakfast? Around 10 am?"

"Yeah, that's not too early," she answered. "I like my Saturday morning lie-in."

"Perfect. I have the gym at nine so I'll shower there and meet you at the Coffee Dock at ten."

I made my way around the table and gave everyone a goodbye hug and kiss, then slowly walked towards the front door.

"Text me when you get home pet," said my mum as usual. I promised her I would.

As I hobbled towards my car, I noticed Michael Lawlor pulling into the driveway. I waited for the family to get out and went to say hello.

"Hey guys. So, you all here to celebrate Gary's birthday and eat cake?"

"Just the young lady I was looking for!" Jake's Mum shouted.

"What did I do now, Mary?" I asked as I gave her a big hug.

"You did nothing, my love. I just wanted to let you know that I passed your number onto a friend of mine whose daughter is getting

116

married. They are looking for someone to write a song for their wedding and I thought of you."

I looked at her, completely puzzled.

"Why did you think of me?

"Michelle, don't be so silly. It's your thing and they will pay you. Come on hun. Go for it."

"Yeah Shell, this might make you rich. Just think of the number of people who would love to have their very own, specially written wedding song?" Michael piped up as he greeted me with a hug too.

"Cha-Ching!" added Sam, as she waited for Michael to finish so she could give me a hug as well.

"Okay, I suppose I can meet with them and see. Thanks for thinking of me, Mary. So, who are they?"

"It's my friend Geraldine's daughter. You wouldn't know them. They are from Churchfield. I'll be going to the wedding myself, Shell, so we can go together."

"When is it?"

"Next Saturday."

"What?! Seriously, Mary! Who do you think I am? Andrew Lloyd Webber?!"

Michael laughed out loud and Sam hit him to shut him up.

"Well, they only decided a few days ago they wanted their own song so they'd only just started to look for someone to write it. They'll probably call you tomorrow."

I was too tired to argue. I nodded in agreement and limped to the car.

"What happened to you, Shell?" Sam asked.

"I joined a gym. That's what happened to me."

Michael laughed out loud again and Sam slapped him again. I sat in the car and put the window down to speak to Mary.

"I'll call over tomorrow night if you're around?"

"I'll be there," she said. "Drive safely now."

"I will. Enjoy your night, guys."

"See ya tomorrow night Shell," said Mike. "A bath in Epsom salts will sort out your muscles!"

"Cheers Mike."

When I arrived home I texted Mum and filled a bath. After I had soaked for a while, I dried off and slipped into bed, all nice and relaxed. I didn't even notice myself falling asleep.

"I feel your pain Shell, I really do. But no pain, no gain," Jake said as he lay next to me in the bed.

"No kidding!" I answered. "Now you tell me!"

"Well done, though," he said, still lying there. "I'm very impressed. All this clearing out, The Gym, the gym instructor and now finally back to songwriting. God Shell, I mean your face should be next to the Nike logo. *Just do it!*"

I laughed at Jake in a way that felt so familiar. "I see what you're doing, Jake Lawlor. I know you. You are trying to slip in stuff and make me do this wedding song, aren't you?"

"Do you remember how I mentioned that there might be areas of your life that you might want to improve or work on?"

"Yes?"

"Well, I'm going to give you a great way to do that...and help you put some fun and excitement back into your life. You're going to do a bucket list."

"Oh? Okay."

"101 things to do while you are alive. Or, as I like to put it, 101 things to do to make you *feel* alive. I did loads off my list but I never got to the end due to unforeseen circumstances. Being dead is a bit of a setback."

"Yeah, no kidding," I agreed. "How many had you done?"

"Seventy-five," he replied immediately.

"Wow, really? That many?"

"Yup! I would have had the first list of 101 done by 40 at the rate I was going."

"Wow! That's amazing, Jake. I can guess some of them but tell me them anyway?"

"Sure, I'll share a few of mine, but whatever you put on yours, be certain you want to do it because it's for you, not for show, okay?"

"Yeah, Jake. I know it's not for show. I get ya."

"Well Michelle, I have; Been on safari in Africa; Learned to swim; Ridden in a hot-air balloon; learned Spanish; earned a degree; fought in a Thai boxing match; organised a fundraiser; climbed Machu Picchu in Peru; been to the Bahamas; I've been on the radio; run a

119

marathon; cycled the Ring of Kerry; written a newspaper column; petted tigers in Thailand; been on TV; been rock climbing; zorbing in New Zealand; zip-lined; learned yoga; taken my mum to see New York; driven my dream car; been skydiving; signed up to be an organ donor; explored Rome - and seen the Pope; learned how to do a cart-wheel; learned to play the guitar; seen Paris from the top of the Eiffel Tower; bungee jumped; climbed Carrauntoohil; walked the Camino; swam with dolphins; completed a triathlon; learned how to ice skate; learned how to ski; seen the Giant's Causeway; met the Dalai Lama; completed a photography course; read over 500 books; walked in the Grand Canyon; I've been sandboarding; driven a dune buggy; learned how to do a poi dance; learned how to *breakdance*; learned how to do a headstand and a handstand; seen Old Trafford; shot a rifle; walked the strip in Las Vegas; driven a Formula One car; been to Madison Square Garden; travelled on the Orient Express; learned how to speed skip; been in the audience on *Top Gear*; held a snake; fed a shark; sailed a yacht; been Player Of The Year for the soccer club; I've been to a Tony Robbins seminar; completed the Artist's Way course; invented something cool; been on a blind date; learned how to play the piano; learned how to play the harmonica; trained a football team; learned archery; I've been to the Galway Races; I've seen the Northern Lights; I've gone night kayaking; learned sign language; trekked through a jungle; entered a bodybuilding competition and been a 'people millionaire'."

I'm not sure which was more impressive; the list itself or the fact that he could remember all of that.

120

"That's a heck of a list," I said. "I'll definitely have to rob a few of your ideas. I like the sound of the hot air balloon or going to the Bahamas!"

"That's great Shell, but what else do you really want to do?"

"I hadn't really thought about it," I said, truthfully.

"Well," he replied, "this is as good a time as any to start thinking about it. Come up with a few now."

"Um...ok." I thought for a moment. "I'd like to get into better shape."

"Good. Be more specific!"

"Okay: I want to be a size 10 and weigh 10 stone."

"Better. Keep going."

"I want to go horse riding. I've never been and I always wanted to."

"Good Shell. Just keep thinking like that; no restrictions. Go mad."

"Okay, I want to visit Canada, Hawaii, France and Italy. I want to learn a martial art. I want to visit Westport in County Mayo and climb Croagh Patrick. I want to...I want to...." I paused and tried to think of more.

"Think about your work," Jake said. "Is it where you want to be? Are you doing what you love?"

"I want to find a job I love. I want to write a new song, I want to ask Ivan out on a date, I want to....."

"Hold up, Shell!" Jake stopped me mid flow. "Did I just hear you say you want to ask a boy out?"

"Yes, you did and I do, but I don't think I have the guts to do it."

"Shelly this is perfect. It's the perfect opportunity to start your list and to get a feel for ticking things off! So for you, it's asking a guy on a date for the first time ever; write a wedding song in a week..."

I held up my hand and he stopped mid-sentence.

"There you go again, Jake. No pushing, remember? You said it should be stuff I want to do!"

"Well Shell, you did say ask Ivan out on a date and I know you want to write again. Who are you kidding? It's your passion! I really never understood why you stopped."

I look at him, trying to think of a reason. I took a deep breath. There was no reason.

"You're right," I admitted. "I do want to."

Jake smiled.

"Good for you Shell, that's the hardest part over."

"What do you mean the hardest part? I still have to ask Ivan out! Cringe! And, I have to write an amazing song in a week. No pressure."

"The hardest part is always making the decision. Now, it's just the action, and in fairness, you've become really good at that."

"Any tips on asking him out?"

"Well, he's single so that's a help."

"What? How do you know that?"

Jake looked at me with his "are you seriously asking me?" face on.

"Right," I said. "Dead. Know everything. Of course."

"Okay, Shell. Firstly, I know Ivan from way back when I dated Nicky and I know he has a type. You fit the description."

"I do?"

"Well, you're breathing!" Jake laughed. I was not impressed.

"I'm kidding," he said, relenting. "You're good looking, tall, blonde, cute, and a little bit naïve."

"Thanks, I think."

"I think you should suss him out tomorrow. Ask him about his hobbies and interests, and be interested in what he says. Get details that you'll remember the next time you meet him. Ask if he's doing anything exciting over the weekend. Find out stuff you can use to chat the next time you meet."

"That's it? That's your great romantic advice, Don Juan?"

"Ha ha, Shell. Yes! It is, actually, and trust me: it's your foundation. You gotta put in the work. You'll only reap what you sow."

"Yes, well...let's talk about reaping Ivan next time. What about the song? I only have a week! What do you think I should do?"

"First things first," was the reply. "Tomorrow, you start your list. At the top write a song in a week; number two, ask a man out on a date. Then follow your list! Write the song first and ask Ivan out second. Got it? Rome wasn't built in a day but a bit of it was. Just focus on one thing until it's done and then move to the next. By the time you have the song written and it's time to ask Ivan out, we'll have the perfect plan for the asking and for the date and for whatever else comes your way."

"Fair enough," I conceded. "I have enough to deal with, with this song, so I can afford to be patient."

"Shell, nearly that time again. I have to go."

I remembered, at long last, that I needed to ask him something before I awoke.

"Jake! Wait! Don't go yet! What's the story with *Galileo*? The song! I know you love it but why do I keep hearing it?"

He smiled and looked thoughtful.

"I can't tell you yet, but I will. I promise."

I felt impatient, but I trusted him. I started to tell him that I'd wait for his explanation, but he was already gone and I was awake.

*Chapter 11 - Sleep 11*

*Saturday 2nd November*

As I opened my eyes, I felt the warm sun on my face. It beamed in my bedroom window. I turned over in the bed to shield my eyes from the bright rays shining in on me.

I stretched my body across my bed, trying to gauge if there was still pain from yesterday's workout. The Epsom salts bath seemed to have worked. That was a relief. I walked to the dresser at the other side of the room and grabbed a pen and notepad before sitting at my desk and writing at the top of the page in large letters; '101 Things To Do While Alive', with the numbers 1 to 101 down the side margin.

1. Write a love song in less than a week.

2. Ask Ivan out on a date.

After sitting staring at my nascent list for a while I finally got up and got ready to go to the gym. Just as I was parking my car, my phone rang; it was an unknown number.

"Hello?"

"Hello, is that Michelle Morrissey?" The voice at the other end asked.

"Yes, speaking."

"Oh great! My name is Tracy. My Mum, Geraldine, is friends with Mary Lawlor and she passed on your number. She said you might be able to help us out with a wedding song. I really hope you can!"

"I'll do my best, Tracy! The wedding is next weekend, yeah?"

"Yes, next Saturday. But, I have faith it will all work out. We just thought that it would be an original idea and I've heard you're brilliant."

"Oh, well thanks, Tracey."

"Could you meet us today to have a chat?" she asked. "I presume you'll need to know a bit about us if you are going to write a song for us. And, of course, we can go through other details like payment and arrangements for the day."

"Yeah, I can do that," I said. "What time?"

"One o'clock at the Lake View Hotel? We can meet you at the bar?"

"Perfect! I'll be there. I'll sit at the bar waiting so you know where to look for me."

"That's great, Michelle!" she said excitedly. "Thanks a million, we're looking forward to meeting you."

As I put down the phone, I noticed Ivan getting out of his car. I decided to seize the opportunity, grabbed my gear bag and walked towards him.

"Morning, Shelly!" he greeted me. "How are the legs?"

"I was crippled yesterday," I laughed. "It really snuck up on me but, last night I had a bath with Epsom salts and I feel fine today."

126

"Good old Epsom salts!" he said with a smile. "They should be by every bathtub. You might need them again later, though. I'll be training you today and its arms day. If you felt the legs, you'll certainly feel the arms!"

That sounded a little intimidating, but it was as good a place as any to strike up some sort of rapport.

"So," I said, "is being sadistic a requirement to work here?"

He laughed.

"Oh yeah, of course! Along with being good looking."

"And modest," I added.

"And modest. You've got to have good looking trainers for the good looking clients. It's just good business sense."

I giggled like a schoolgirl and felt myself starting to blush, so I quickly walked ahead of him and into the changing rooms. I sat down and had a little pep talk with myself, "Okay, Michelle, take it slow and don't get too excited. All you need to do is stick to the plan like Jake said. Get out there and be fabulous."

I walked into The Gym and over to the corner where Ivan was setting things up for me, then he asked me a question that really surprised me:

"Are you doing anything exciting for the weekend?"

My heart skipped a beat. What was happening?

"Em," I burbled, trying not to gush, and composed myself as best I could. "Me? No. Nothing too exciting. Just going to visit some friends tonight and attempting to write a song."

127

"You're writing a song?" he said, with a bemused look on his face.

"Yeah. I have gotten roped into writing a wedding song last minute for a friend of a friend's daughter's wedding. Oh, and it's next week, so, ya know! No pressure!"

He seemed genuinely impressed.

"Wow, that's pretty cool. Do you sing?"

"Well, it comes in handy when someone wants to hear the song you wrote!" I cringed inside and told myself to resist the urge to be a smarty-pants.

"Sarcasm suits you!" he mocked, gently. "That's pretty cool, though. I like a girl who can sing. It's very attractive."

This seemed to be going well. I decided to take control of the chat.

"So...um...are you doing anything exciting over the weekend yourself?"

"Working today, heading to Offaly tonight. A few of us are going to do a parachute jump tomorrow."

"Now that's cool; slightly crazy but cool. Is it something you always do? Are you an extremist?"

"Oh no, I have only done it once before for charity. This time it's just for fun. I suppose I like doing new stuff, you know? A break from the norm? There's a group of us who go cycling together regularly and one of the guys is getting married next Saturday. His best man organised for us to go out in Offaly tonight for the stag and to do the jump tomorrow morning."

"Wow! Good idea for a stag. Jump out of a plane, hung over."

"Yeah I know!" he laughed. "It'll go down well in the wedding speeches! Actually, I reckon Seán is only doing this so he has material for his best man speech."

Ivan looked at his watch.

"We better get you trained."

It was far from easy, and I realised that I wasn't as strong as I thought I was, but Ivan was there all the way, encouraging me and keeping a close eye on my technique. By the time we got through the session, my arms were like jelly. I went back to the changing room, had a quick shower, and fumbled with my clothes with my uncooperative, quivering arms. When I was leaving, Ivan was meeting another client. He asked me when I planned on coming back in and I said it'd be before work on Monday. He smiled his big smile.

"Good luck with the song. Can't wait for you to sing it to me."

"Thanks. Good luck with the jump!"

I watched him walk back into the gym, just barely managed to stop myself from behaving like one of the girls in the Diet Coke ads, and called Eve to make sure we were still meeting.

As I drove from The Gym to the Coffee Dock, I thought of how easy it was to talk to Ivan. There was definitely a spark there. I was amazed at how he asked me all the right questions. It made it effortless.

It was almost like he knew and everything fitted perfectly together. A song I liked was playing on the radio, so I turned it up and sang along.

I thought about how there seemed to be a lovely flow to things at the moment. I had never experienced this before; at least not that I was aware of. When I arrived at the car park of the Coffee Dock, Eve was sitting inside by the window in the usual seat.

"Good morning, little sister."

"Good morning, big sister."

"How was The Gym?"

"Oh, my Buddha, Eve! Why didn't you tell me about Ivan? Delish, with a taste of more."

"Ha! I didn't even think about it! So, I take it you like?"

"Hell yeah!" I practically shouted. "He's perfect! He's fit and friendly...a rare breed."

"Oh Michelle you crack me up, I think he's single too, so that's good."

"He is!" I blurted out, without thinking.

"Okay, Sherlock Holmes," she mocked. "You did your homework. Were you stalking him on Facebook already?"

"Yes, and I am going to have him. That's all there is to it. I'm going to ask him out." That got her attention. I'd never asked a guy out in my life.

"What? Are you crazy? You're going to ask a guy out?!" she laughed.

"It's the second thing on my bucket list."

130

"You have a bucket list?"

"Yeah! I started one this morning and asking a guy out...well, asking *Ivan* out, is number two, right after 'write a song in a week'."

"I don't know what's got such a fire under your ass, but I'm enjoying watching you in action."

"You ain't seen nothing yet" I promised her, and we both burst out into laughter.

We chatted over breakfast about the song I had to write, then we talked about Ivan some more. I gave her a blow-by-blow account of our chat in The Gym. After lots of coffee and lots of gossip, I dropped Eve home and went home to start setting up for my songwriting session.

It had been a while since I had played, so the guitar was out of tune. I was a singer in a band called 'The Dreamers' – me, Claire, Fran, Alan and Ross. We played around the local pubs on the long weekends but mainly we performed at weddings. Each of us had a full-time job, so we did it for extra cash and, more importantly, for the love of music. Since joining the group, I had stopped playing my own music and hadn't been playing any guitar.

By the time I got everything set up, it was time to go to meet the bride and groom-to-be. The Lake View Hotel is probably one of the poshest hotels in the country. It's a five-star hotel; luxurious bedrooms, modern state-of-the-art gym, modern conference facilities and an award winning Swedish spa. I had performed there last year with the band for a wedding that had three bands and a DJ throughout the day and night. The place was top class.

131

As I sat at the bar, I wondered what questions I ought to ask. How did ye meet? Describe yourselves? Or maybe I should just let them to all the talking.

As I was deep in thought, I heard a voice from behind me; "Michelle?"

I turned to be greeted by two smiling faces. "Yes!" I said, "but you can call me Shelly."

"Shelly, I'm Tracey, and this is my fiancé, Aaron."

I reached out to shake Aaron's hand.

"Pleasure to meet you, Shelly, we are really excited about this!" he said with a big smile. "Would you like a drink?"

"No, thank you," I told him. "I'm fine with just water."

Tracey and I took a seat while Aaron went to the bar to order a white wine for her, and we started to make light conversation.

"It's so nice to have a glass of wine in the middle of the day," she giggled. "I feel like I'm on holidays. Aaron has to drive to Offaly later with the boys for his stag party, so I get to be an alcoholic.

"I've heard great things about your music, my mum said that Mary told her your band is fabulous. We're so excited! We just couldn't pick a song for our first dance and you hear so much about first dance songs. I mean..."

As Tracey kept talking, I couldn't stop thinking what a coincidence. Were Aaron and Ivan friends? What were the chances that the one guy I fancy is going to be at the wedding where I have to sing the song I have a week to write?

132

Tracey was a petite woman in her late twenties with dark shoulder-length hair, large brown eyes and a beautiful smile. When Aaron joined us, she was still talking. I don't think she'd taken a breath since she started her first sentence. Aaron placed Tracey's drink on the table and sat down next to her. As she lifted her glass to take a drink and a breath, he took her other hand in his. "I can write about that," I thought to myself.

"So what do you need to know, Shelly? I mean, as Tracey probably told you, we only decided this last minute but we feel it's right and we're both excited to break the norm. We have a band for the wedding, 'Aces and Stars.' Do you know them?"

"Yeah, they're great," I replied. "How did you get them? I thought they only played during the summer. From what I hear, they work for four months flat and take the rest of the year off because they make so much."

Aaron laughed, "Yeah, you're right, but my younger brother plays lead guitar with them."

Tracey grabbed Aaron's arm lovingly and added "he's only 22 years old and the job gets him through college. He's studying to be a doctor."

Aaron smiled at Tracey and placed a kiss on her cheek.

"It's all about who you know," I said with a grin.

"It sure is! He has offered to accompany you, or you can bring your own musician. Up to you, just let us know what you need."

That could be interesting, I decided.

133

"Okay, that's great thanks. I am not too sure of the details yet, till I write the song, of course! Where is the wedding on and what time do you need me there? When can I practice with the sound equipment?"

Tracey took over again, and Aaron happily lets her.

"It's on here, and you're welcome to attend the whole wedding. You can come with Mary if you want. The stage will be set up the night before, so you can practice that morning or before we arrive back here in the evening, up to you. Also, if you need anything else, like a dress or shoes, I can have it arranged!"

Aaron looked at straight at me, "We know it's a bit of pressure but we just want something original. We're just two people who are happy and want to look back on the day with happy memories. Does that help?"

"I can see that," I reassured them, "and it does, thanks."

We chatted for another while, discussing details and payment. I told them I wouldn't know how much to charge until I figured out how long it would take me to write and rehearse, as well as to perform, which they were happy to hear. The conversation flowed nicely. Before too long, though, Aaron checked the time on his phone.

"I have to make tracks soon," he announced. "I have a stag to attend!"

Aaron was a tall man. Next to his wife-to-be, he was like a giant. He was quite shallow, with dark, tightly cut hair and piercing blue eyes: a very attractive man. I thought they were well matched. We gathered our bits and pieces and walked out of the hotel and into the car park.

134

I watched them walk to their car with linked arms. Aaron opened the car door for Tracey and I was lost in thought as they drove off. They seemed so happy and so in love. As I sat into my car and turned the key in the ignition, I remembered my earlier lesson from Jake: over-thinking makes everything harder. I decided to not worry or stress about the song and just go home and write it.

Armed with tea and a sandwich, I set myself up in my little work area, trying out a few chords and humming a melody. As I did, I thought about my Mum and Dad dancing around the living room when we were kids. I recalled Cara and her husband Kevin's first dance at their wedding. I drifted back to Tracey and Aaron; how the love and happiness shone out of them. That did the trick. The words just flowed, as if out of nowhere. I began to sing. Before I knew it, I had written two verses and the chorus.

"Bravo, Maestro" I murmured to myself. I glanced at the clock; it was 4.30 pm. I felt tired and was starting to feel sore all over. I threw myself on the sofa and fell fast asleep.

"'Bravo Maestro' is right," Jake said enthusiastically. "You've surprised me!"

"Well, what can I say Jake? I'm a genius."

"Shell, everyone is a genius but not everyone uses it. So, how do you feel? I mean that's one off the list already!"

"Super, Jake. I feel super! I have a dilemma, though. How do I charge them for the song? It only took me two hours to write. What should I do?"

135

"Well, Shell. That depends on the value you put on what you have created and the value they put on owning their own song."

"That's a good way to look at it," I agreed. "I could say that I'll sleep on it but I already kind of am."

"Don't worry," Jake said reassuringly. "You'll know what to charge by Monday, or the universe will take the decision out of your hands. Sometimes synchronicity solves all!"

"What the heck is synchronicity?" I asked with a raised eyebrow.

"Coincidence!" Jake answered. "You know, like when you think of someone and then they call you? Or, you think of a song and it comes on the radio. It's when things are in sync. Not by mistake or by accident, but in harmony and on purpose."

"That's a nice way of putting it," I said. "I think I had a day like that yesterday."

"You know when it happens because it feels right," he continued, but let's leave that discussion for a while. Today is about number two on your list; asking Ivan out."

"Give me a break, Jake. I'm not Wonder Woman."

"No, Shell, you're not. You're Superwoman, and you're going to take on your next goal with the same attitude as your first!"

"Attitude? I think you mean luck!"

"Actually yes; luck happens when you are prepared and an opportunity arises. Today you were organised and prepared, and then you wrote a song in two hours. If you had never done this before and you didn't have the tools, experience and talent, the result might have been a little different. So on Monday, you'll do the same. You'll do a little homework and you'll have a plan."

"Homework?"

"What have you learned about Ivan in the past two days?"

"Well...he's single. He likes activities that are new, fun and challenging – maybe he's a bit of a thrill-seeker? I think, anyway. He's at his friend's stag for the weekend and they're going to do a parachute jump. His friend happens to be the groom I'm writing the song about, and Ivan will be at the wedding when I sing it."

Jake nodded as if to say "exactly – don't you get it?"

"In that case, you have a topic to discuss with Ivan on Monday morning," he explained. "You have feedback to give him about the song, and a common event to look forward to and discuss. And, very importantly, he did say he thinks a girl who can sing is very attractive."

"But..."

"No buts Shell. And, finally, you have a brilliant date to bring him on and the best part is it's a surprise. You'll blow him away."

"A brilliant date and a surprise?" I was puzzled. "Explain!"

"Remember my ex, Mary?"

"Jake, you were only going out with her a few months ago. Of course, I remember her."

"Yeah, well, you know what I mean. She was awesome and we had a really good relationship. In fact, I would go so far as to say it was the best relationship I had in my life."

"Why did ye split, Jake? I couldn't figure it out."

"She wanted to go travelling and be free and easy and I was ready to start laying the foundations for a different future. We were looking for different things. I believe now that we parted for a reason. But we had a tradition while we were together which we both absolutely loved, and it'll work wonders for you."

I looked at him quizzically.

"Surprise date!" he said. "You take a turn at arranging a date for you and your partner. The person organising it does all the work, all planning, all the paying, and the other person just shows up where and when they're told to."

"Nice idea," I said, "but it sounds like a bit of work."

"Well that's the best part: you're only doing it six times a year. The other six you get to look forward to and just enjoy it. Coming up with ideas and organising it is fun! It really keeps things fresh. Most couples lose what got them excited in the first place; dating, getting to know each other, sharing new experiences and having fun."

"God, that's so true Jake. You might be onto something here."

"I know!" he said. No false modesty for Jake.

"So...you have a suggestion, right?"

"One of the dates I took Mary on was to West Cork for a night. I told her to pack for an overnight stay and an activity. I told her we were leaving and I advised her to bring warm clothes, even though it was summer. She didn't have a clue and the whole way there she tried to

138

guess. It was worth it for the look on her face alone when she found out what we were doing!"

"So what was it, Jake?"

"Night kayaking, off Reen Pier. Mary was blown away. Said it was her best date ever."

That sounded very promising.

"Can you do it all year?"

"Of course!" said Jake. "And tomorrow, you're going to call and enquire about it for you and Ivan."

"But what if he doesn't want to go out with me?"

Jake sighed with exasperation.

"Have you been listening to me at all? To win you must expect to win. Plan B distracts from plan A! Do you get me?"

"Okay okay!" I admitted defeat. "I'll call first thing! How do you reckon I should ask him out?"

"I'm pretty sure you will figure that one out yourself. I mean, do I have to do everything?"

"I suppose I can depend on synchronicity to guide me," I teased, just as I heard a strange sound. I looked around the room, confused.

"What's that noise, Jake?"

*Chapter 12 - Sleep 12*

*Saturday, 2nd November*


I woke on the couch, to the sound of my mobile ringing. I reached over to my keyboard and grabbed the phone.

"Hello?" I said groggily. It was Sam.

"Hey Shell, Mum asked me to phone you to check what time you are calling over, and if you want one of us to collect you so you can have a drink?"

"Oh, that would be sweet, Sam. Are you having a drink too?"

"Does the pope wear a funny hat Shell? I'm a bar manager who's off on a weekend night. Hell yeah, I'm drinking! But I'll be heading into the city later to meet some of my friends, so I won't be here for the night. Just till about 11 pm, if you want to get a lift home in the cab when I am heading off?"

I looked at the clock, it was 7 pm. "Perfect. If one of you can collect me, I can be ready in half an hour. Is Mike around?"

"No, he's off out with Stephanie for dinner and cinema. I can pick you up before I have a drink."

"Great thanks, I'll get ready so. See you soon."

I had a quick shower, changed my clothes and grabbed a wrap for dinner. I noticed that my arms were stiff and sore as I pulled a bottle of wine out of the fridge. While I was frowning and trying to shake some looseness into them, Sam pulled up outside and gave me a missed call. I popped the wine into my bag and went out to meet her.

"Hey Sam, how are you?"

"Great! Going to have this nice quiet start and, then, a wild ending I expect. You?"

"Good for you!" I said with a smile. "I'll probably be home in bed by midnight."

Sam gave me a devilish grin.

"You're more than welcome to join me for a wild night out on the town," she said, wiggling her eyebrows.

"Oh, no thanks. Not my scene at the moment."

"Too cool for Cork?" she teased.

"Hardly! I'm not too cool for anything at the moment!"

"Are you serious?" Sam retorted. "I think you are so cool!"

I laughed it off, but she looked at me earnestly.

"You are! Lots of people think so! Remember my friend, Harry, from Scotland?"

"Yeah, what about him?"

"He thinks you are divine. He always asks about you." Sam attempted to do a Scottish accent, "How's your brother's hot singer friend, eh? I am going to marry her, you know!" I hadn't been expecting that at all.

"What? Are you serious?"

"Yeah, and he's hot and all the girls like him! He could have anyone and he always goes on about you; 'Hot Singer Chick this' and 'Hot Singer Chick' that!"

I think I blushed.

"That's so sweet! Thanks for telling me, Sam."

"That's not all either, Shell," Sam continued, warming to her theme. "There's a few of the regular lads in the bar, and a lot of friends of Jake's, who would definitely go there if they thought they had a shot. You *are* the sexy singer chick. You're a blonde bombshell!"

"Are you winding me up?" I asked suspiciously.

"No! They would totally ask you out! It's just you normally wouldn't be the most approachable girl."

"Yeah, I know. I'm working on it."

"I can see that," she said, and then her tone changed. "How are you getting on, though? I mean, with Jake gone and all?"

"God, shouldn't I be asking *you* that? I suppose, I still feel he's with me. That helps. I know losing him has given me a greater appreciation of life and now I want to live a life that's full of fun and excitement. You know what I mean?"

"I do. I really do. If I learned anything from my big brother, it's to live life to the fullest. Only for Jake, I wouldn't have the confidence and drive I have. I will always be grateful to him, and in a way, I feel he's with me too."

Sam smiled and we drove to the off-license in comfortable silence. As we entered, a voice boomed out in a broad Scottish accent.

142

"Hey, hey! What are you lovely ladies up to this fine evening?"

It was Harry. Sam laughed at the coincidence as I blushed yet again.

"We're off to drink some fine wine in some fine company. You?"

Sam and Harry nattered away for a minute as I stood there, smiling shyly and trying not to make too much eye contact with him. She arranged to meet him at a club later that night, he said goodbye to us both with a huge grin and headed off on his way.

I turned to Sam and laughed.

"What are the chances, eh?"

"Synchronicity at its best," she said.

We grabbed a few bottles of wine, one for Mary, one for Sam and one for the house, as tradition stated. We arrived at the Lawlor house and Mary was sitting in the living room watching *The Late Late Show*.

"Hey, girls. What took you so long? I could have made my own wine while I was waiting for you!"

We laughed at Mary's witty comment. I leant down to the couch where she was sitting to give her a hug and a kiss.

"I hear you are going to do the song for Tracy," she said.

"Yes. I am actually, Mary."

"Isn't she so sweet? And her fella's a dote. Are you coming with me to the whole thing, so?"

"Em, I don't know what to do yet" I replied truthfully. "I might just go to the Afters a bit early to set up and have a rehearsal. I'll let you know."

143

"Have you started the song yet?" Mary asked me.

"One week to write a song. Can it be done? Or will our heroine crash and burn?" Sam asked dramatically.

"Yes, it can be done and it has been done! In fact, it can be done in a day."

"What? A day? Really, Shell?" Sam asked in amazement.

"Yeah, it can. I did it today."

Sam and Mary sat forward in their seats, with looks of disbelief on their faces. "I did it today after meeting Tracey and Aaron. I was inspired."

"See, Shell?" Sam said; "I told you were cool! Will you sing us some?"

"I can't. It's written for the bride and groom and I think they should be the first to hear it. As long as they like it, then I'll sing it at the wedding and they can buy it if they want. Well, that's the plan."

"That's fantastic, Shell!" Mary said as she gave me a hug. "I told you! I knew you could do it. I remember as a young girl before you could even play the piano, you would make up songs and sing them to all of us. Even at such a young age, you had a gift."

"What was the song you wrote for your secondary school graduation mass?" Sam asked.

"Oh, yeah, I'd forgotten about that! It was called 'See ya later.'"

Sam started to sing it. "Don't say goodbye, say see ya later, See ya later...'" I was impressed that she seemed to remember it better than I did.

"Yeah! That was it Sam." It evoked a lot of old memories I'd forgotten I'd had. Mary laughed.

"You might be on *The Late Late Show* singing your song some night and we'll be watching you saying 'I remember when she wrote that! One day, only one day it took her! She had a week, but she only needed one day.'"

We all had a good old chuckle at the thought. We sat, drank wine and talked for hours. After a bit, Sam announced it was time for her to get ready to go out, "I will be 20 minutes and I'm going to call a taxi if you want a lift home Shell?"

I looked over at Mary who looked like she could fall asleep at any minute and accepted the offer. I wanted to record that song properly the following day so I can meet the bride and groom with it on Monday.

"Yes, please," I said to Sam. "Early to bed, early to rise and all that,"

"That's right pet," Mary sat up. "And I'm exhausted."

"Head off to bed," I told her.

"I will," she replied, and then she looked at me with a serious expression.

"Are you alright, Shell?" All of a sudden she sounded very concerned.

I told her I was great and she could tell I was wondering why she'd asked. "Oh, I just wonder how you are since he is gone, you know. I miss him so much..."

Mary started to cry. I jumped up out of my seat and over to console her.

"I know you miss him. I do too. It's just one of these things we have to get through. It'll get easier."

"I know Shell but right now it's hard. I would give anything to just see him once. To just hear his voice, to just feel him in my arms. Anything. I'd give anything." I squeezed her as she sobbed.

"I know, Mary. I know. Tonight when you go to bed, ask him to give you a sign. Tell him you need his help. I think he'll hear you."

"That's a nice idea, Shelly," she sniffled. "Thanks, hun."

I asked her if she wanted me to stay the night.

"No, no, really I'm fine. Thank you. It's just the drinks, you know. They made me a little emotional. But I'm so very proud of you, and you're handling this very well. Jake would be proud of you, too." I smiled a little private smile. I knew he was.

"Thanks, Mary. I appreciate that."

"I'm going to go to bed, I think. Don't tell Sam I was upset. She'll only worry. Okay?"

I gave her a long hug and swore I wouldn't breathe a word to Sam, and she kissed me on the cheek and squeezed my hand before she headed up the stairs, shouting "night night" to Sam as she passed her bedroom door.

As I waited for Sam, I walked around the living room looking at the pictures of all of the kids from both families when we were really young, all the way up to Christmas 2010 when Mary made us all stand in for a picture together out in the back garden in the snow. As I look around, I started to feel a little nostalgic. It was the first time since Jake passed, apart from the morning of the funeral, that I felt sad. I realised that Jake's visits weren't going to be forever. It was just for now. And, after my 21$^{st}$ sleep, I wouldn't see Jake in person again. It would just be those pictures and I would not hear his voice again or feel his warm comforting hugs.

Sam interrupted my thoughts, clomping down the stairs to tell me the taxi was waiting outside. As we were on the way to my house she did her best to convince me to go dancing.

"Are you sure you don't want to come, Shell? Last chance...there'll be boys!"

I laughed at her choice of temptation, but I was adamant that I was going to go home. I closed the door of the taxi, walked up the pathway to my house, opened the front door and took a moment to appreciate the peace and quiet. I didn't even turn on the lights. I just walked straight upstairs, undressed and hopped into bed. I was out like a light.

"Just before we start, Jake, I have to ask you something."

"How did you get a word in before me? You're getting good at this!" Jake said, with a look of pride on his face.

"Can you use one of these sleeps to visit your Mum?"

For just a moment he looked sad and vulnerable.

"No," he answered softly.

"Why not? You can give her one of mine!"

147

"It doesn't work like that, Shell. Just you. Just 21 times. That's the deal."

"She really needs you," I told him.

"My mother doesn't need me," he said, "and if she did, I'd have gone to her. Mum's been through hard times in her life. She's a tough cookie. Life…" for once, Jake seemed a little lost for words. "Life has taught her enough to bring her through any challenge. She's only human. She has moments when she feels sad, happy, mad, angry, jealous, loving, caring and all the other emotions that we humans experience. But, I can tell you truthfully: she doesn't need anyone."

"Okay. I'm sorry I asked. It's just…when I saw her upset tonight I wanted to help. The only way I knew how was for you to visit her."

"I know you meant well, Shell. Don't worry. She'll feel a lot better in the morning and you never know; the suggestion you made might mean pleasant dreams. Synchronicity, you know?"

"For something I'd never thought about before, it's been cropping up a lot today," I told him.

"It happens every day," said Jake. "You're just aware of it now. I always loved the idea. I much prefer to believe that a coincidental event or experience happened for a reason and has a meaning rather than believe that it's totally random. Does that make sense?"

"Yeah, totally. I mean it doesn't harm anyone really, does it?"

"That's the best part. Just like anything you think that makes you feel good, it doesn't matter what anyone else thinks. If you are being the good gardener in your mind and having good thoughts, you'll feel good. When you feel good, more good thoughts will come. That's the simplicity of synchronicity, Shelly. In the words of Albert Einstein, 'everything should be made as simple as possible...but not simpler.' He really got it."

"Got what?"

"Life, Shell! He got the purpose of life."

"I always thought he was more about science and logic than philosophy," I said.

"Logic will get you from A to B, Shell. Imagination will take you everywhere," was Jake's reply

"Oh, I like that one. Who said that?"

"Albert Einstein!" Jake laughed. I laughed too.

"He was a pretty smart guy after all!" I joked.

"He was," Jake agreed, "and he knew we're all geniuses, even if we don't see it. He also said 'if you judge a fish on its ability to climb a tree, it will live its whole life believing that it is stupid'." That one really appealed to me.

"I wish I'd known that quote in school," I said. "It would have been handy in maths class. It's true, though, isn't it? We beat ourselves up when we're not so good at something and we end up feeling awful. We should focus on what we do well in order to feel good."

"Nicely put," Jake nodded. "And, while on the subject of doing things well, good job on writing that song so quickly!"

"Thanks, Jake! By any chance, did you have anything to do with it?"

"Shelly, I think you might have the wrong idea here. If I had that kind of power, I would have just had you like a puppet on a string for the rest of your life and I wouldn't have needed to appear to you at all."

"Yeah, I suppose that makes sense."

"Don't give away your genius! You deserve it. That song came from you, and you should be really proud."

"Oh, I am!" I assured him. "I mean I feel really good about it, and it was fun being in that flow. In fact, it was familiar. I remember when we were kids and I felt hurt or sad or scared, I found writing a song would take me away from it. It was like I released the emotion into the song. Does that make sense?"

"That's probably what was happening."

"Probably. But today was different. It was already a good emotion, and by the end, it was better. I felt the love. Kind of corny eh?"

"Totally corny! But I understand."

"And what a coincidence that Aaron and Ivan are friends!"

"Coincidence or synchronicity?"

"Synchronicity, then." I laid it on thick, batting my eyelashes and fanning myself exaggeratedly with my hand. "It means that Ivan is the one. He's the man I'm going to marry! He's going to be the father of my children!"

Jake laughed at my silly act. "Yeah, Shell! You are going to have to ask him out first, though!" he said. "So don't forget to call about the kayaking tomorrow."

"I know Jake. I will. Reen Pier, ya?"

"Yes, and after that, all you gotta do is ask him out. Boom! You're going to have to add a few more things to your Bucket List, or you'll run out of goals in no time. Oh, one of them could be to appear on *The Late Late Show*! You could bring Mum. She'd be delighted."

"Sure thing. I'll put it right after 'win the lotto' and just before 'become a supermodel.'" We both got a good laugh out of that one, but when we calmed down again Jake said it was time for him to leave.

"Really?" I asked. "Already?! God, the time together seems like minutes, Jake. It's weird. In fact, the fact that I haven't actually slept in nearly two weeks is hard to even imagine."

"That's because you're getting the sleep, you're just experiencing it differently" he explained. "When you wake up after sleeping normally, even before all of this, it doesn't feel like that long a time, does it?"

"No, that's true. You're right."

"Of course I am," he grinned. "See you tomorrow."

Chapter 13 - Sleep 13

Sunday, 3<sup>rd</sup> November

Sunlight poured through the window illuminating my room. I lay there, basking in it, and stretched. My arms were still very sore. I should have had a bath in Epsom salts before bed.

Slowly, I got out of bed and made my way downstairs, opening the curtains in each room to leave the sunshine in and opening the windows to let some fresh air in. It was another beautiful autumn day and I wanted to enjoy it.

I made my breakfast and sang my newly written song over and over by way of practice. I still had no thoughts on a title, though. I took my cup of coffee, walked over to the keyboard and played the song again while recording it before going through the same routine with the guitar. When I got to recording the vocals, I felt stuck. Something wasn't right. There was something missing. It took a while before I could put my finger on just what it needed, but a sudden flash of inspiration hit me.

"It needs a male vocal!" I said aloud to an empty room. The song should have been a duet from the very start. "Silly Shelly! How did you miss that?"

After spending the morning re-recording the track to give Tracey and Aaron on Monday, I decided to go out to get some air. It was just starting to get a little chill, so, I put on my coat, scarf and gloves and took off for a walk. The area where I live has overlapping trees, and as I walked the leaves were falling all around me, like rain. I soaked in the beauty of the day and wondered if Mary dreamt of Jake last night. I decided to pop over and say good morning.

As I walked up the long driveway of the Lawlor house, I was greeted by Michael and his girlfriend Stephanie. He greeted me with a smile. It was good to see him.

"Hiya Mike!" I said. "We missed you last night. Hey, Stephanie! How are you?"

I leant in and gave them both a hug.

"Yeah, Mum said ye had a nice night," Mike said. "She's in right form this morning for someone who had a bottle of wine last night!"

"She even got up and cooked us all a full Irish breakfast!" Stephanie said with a shocked expression. "We're going to try to walk it off now."

We chatted for another few minutes, then said our goodbyes as they headed out to burn through a few of the full Irish calories.

"Oh, the back door's open, by the way" Michael shouted as they walked off.

As I approached the back door I heard singing from the kitchen. "*Who puts the rainbow in the sky? Who lights the stars at night? Who dreamt up someone so divine? Someone like you and made them mine?*"

*Galileo*, again. Mary was singing. She must have dreamed of Jake.

"Lovely singing, Mar!" I said as I walked in.

Mary jumped, startled, and turned around to greet me.

"Shelly! Good morning, love. Are you hungry? There's plenty of food!"

"Oh God no thanks, Mary. I've had breakfast. What has you so chirpy?"

She looked at me with a big smile.

"Guess who I had a dream about last night?"

"Was it Elvis?" I asked cheekily.

"Smart ass!" Mary laughed. "It was Jake! It was like all dreams but it just meant more. It was as if he came just to give me peace of mind. He was always so open-minded. Once, he went to a talk with his buddy Martin on Esoteric Philosophy, and when he came home that night he told me about it. He always liked the idea that when people died they could send a little message to you in some way."

"Do you believe it Mar?"

She looked pensive, staring into the distance for a moment with her head on one side.

"To be very honest Shelly, I choose to believe it. Jake always said 'your beliefs are for you and my beliefs are for me and as long as they're right for us, we'll never have to defend them or convince anyone of them.' And that I do believe. It feels good to me to believe that there has been a sign sent to me, so by God, I'm going to take that good feeling and enjoy it! We spend far too much time looking at and for the

154

negative. It's so much nicer to appreciate and focus on the positive, isn't it?"

"You're spot on!" I told her. "I'm beginning to see that more now."

"Shelly, there has been a massive change in you since Jake died. And, if you don't mind me saying so because I am going to anyway..."

"Go on Mar."

"Well...we were all starting to think you were in denial. But I can see it now."

"What can you see?"

"While Jake was alive he inspired all of us, but for some reason, Shell, you were always the one he felt he couldn't get to. He often joked that he felt like you hadn't lived enough lives. He loved you but he used to get frustrated at your lack of ambition and, how easily you would give up and give into everything. But since he's gone, you seem to be more alive, more positive. I know he would be proud of you."

"Thanks, Mar," I said. It meant a lot to me to hear her say that. Aware that things were getting a little heavy for that hour of the morning, she changed the subject and offered me a cup of tea. We sat down and drank a cup each.

"You're back into work tomorrow, aren't you?" she asked. "How do you feel about that?"

"I don't mind," I answered truthfully. "I'm going to go to The Gym before work to start my day on a good note, and I'm going to just do

155

my job and get on with it. I can't change the people around me, but I can change how I react to them."

This got the seal of approval from Mary, who ceremoniously poured me another cup of tea.

We drank several more and chatted about working in the hospital. I left at noon and walked back home to get the song finished up for the next day. I wasn't long in the door when my mother rang me.

"We're going to go out for a bite later, your dad and myself. Do you want to join us? Probably around 5 pm or so."

"Oh, I might just do that!" I said. It sounded like a nice thing to do. "Where ye going?"

"Gallagher's. Do you want us to pick you up, so you can have a glass of wine with dinner?"

"Cheers, Mum. That would be nice. I'll see you both at five, so."

"Okay love. 'Bye."

I hung up the phone and went to get my clothes ready for the morning, making my way through a mental list: Training gear. Wash gear. Towels. Work clothes. Makeup. As I got everything ready, I thought about going back to work the next day and of how much easier, more fun and more rewarding it was to write instead. I still had no idea what to charge. How much would someone be willing to pay for their own song at a wedding? Then, a new thought popped into my head, one I had never had before: "what if I just wrote songs for a living?"

I finished getting myself ready for the next day, ran downstairs and pulled out my notepad and a pen.

**The 101 things to do while I am alive:**

No.1 Write a song in a week

No.2 Ask man out on a date (Ivan)

I then started to add more:

No.3 Become a songwriter

No.4 Visit Rome

No.5 Climb the Galtees

No.6 Learn to swim

No.7 Appear on *The Late Late Show*

No.8 Read at least 12 books next year

No.9 Learn to salsa dance

No.10 Get master guitar lessons

I didn't stop until I made it all the way to 101. Then, I sat back in the chair and sighed, feeling proud of myself. It was 4 pm. Time to get ready to meet my parents.

I grabbed the recording I'd made earlier that morning, went back upstairs and popped the CD into my gear bag, then I decided to get properly dressed up for dinner. After all, this was the first opportunity to get done up I'd had in a long time, and you never know who you might meet.

It was just starting to get dark outside when my parents arrived, so I walked around the house closing the curtains and blinds. I left on the hall light and the living room lamps and turned on the timer for the heating, setting it for two hours later so the house would be warm when I

157

arrived back. Then, off out the door, I went. I jumped into the back seat of the car.

"What you been up to?" my mother asked.

"I was at Mary's last night with her and Sam. We had a few drinks. It was a good night. Then I was out for a walk this morning, so I popped into Mary's again for a cuppa. Then I finished up writing that song, I have to let the bride and groom hear it tomorrow."

"You wrote a song, Shell?" Dad piped up.

"I did!" I said proudly. "I wrote a song. It's been a while but I seem to still have it."

"Well done!" he beamed.

"Is that the song for Geraldine's daughter?" asked Mum.

"Yes, but...you're going to have to tell me: who is Geraldine? I can't place her! I thought I knew all the nurses in the hospital."

"Oh she's not a nurse," Mum said. "She's a counsellor, Mary knows her years. They became friends when Mary's Pat got really sick and she was going for counselling. I think they just clicked and, as far as I know, Geraldine's husband died around the same time, so they got to be very close."

"Do you know her?"

"I know her to see. She's only in and out of the hospital once a week. She is one of the hospital counsellor available to staff if they have had a traumatic experience."

We arrived at Gallagher's. Dad drove up to the door and dropped us off and then went to park the car. As Mum and I walked into the bar, she looked me up and down "Look at you all dressed up!" she commented.

"Well, I am going out for dinner. I thought I better put in the effort!" was my retort.

"Oh yes, Michelle! For us, is it?" Mum joked.

We walked into the bar. Sam was working.

"The Morrissey women out on the town!" she declared.

"Just out for a quiet bite!" I told her. "Dad's here too. How was your night afterwards, last night?"

Sam smiled. "It was amazing, thanks. But, sure I always have fun. Even on my own."

Mum laughed. "If you can't enjoy your own company, how can you expect anyone else to enjoy it?"

"Wise words!" Sam agreed.

Dad walked up behind us. "Hello, old man!" Sam greeted him. They had a great relationship and enjoyed having fun at each other's expense.

Dad grinned. "I'm not old," he insisted. "I'm vintage."

We got a white wine each for Mum and me, and Dad ordered a sparkling water. I excused myself to go to the bathroom and as I walked through the bar I heard a voice calling out to me. It was Aaron. He walked over to me.

"How are you doing?"

"Hi, Aaron!" I beamed back. "I'm great, thanks. How was the stag?"

"Oh amazing, thanks! We are just back from Offaly and we decided to finish up with a bite to eat and a few drinks here. So how is the song?"

"Oh, it's done! Ye can hear it tomorrow."

"What, really? Tracey will be thrilled! Are we meeting you tomorrow?"

"Yes, tomorrow evening if possible? That way you both can listen to it and decide if you want to go ahead with everything."

"Super stuff, Shell."

I became aware of someone walking up behind me, and a familiar voice said my name. It was Ivan. I concentrated on not blushing.

"Aaron was just saying what a great time ye had," I said.

"Do you two know each other?" Aaron asked, surprised.

"I was just going to ask the same question!" said Ivan.

I gave up on the struggle not to blush.

"I go to Ivan's gym," I said to Aaron.

"And Shelly is writing a song for Tracey and myself for the wedding," Aaron told Ivan.

"Oh, that's the song you were on about!" Ivan exclaimed. "Wow, small world!"

"Yeah," I said self-consciously. "Tell me about it! But...er...it's lovely talking to you both, but I have to use the ladies and join my family for dinner. So, I'll see you in the morning Ivan, and I'll see you tomorrow evening Aaron?"

"Perfect," Aaron responded.

"See you bright and early!" Ivan said. "You look great, by the way."

I felt him watching me as I walked away and I nearly burst out in a fit of girlish giggles as I entered the ladies. Synchronicity, indeed.

I got back just as we were being seated for dinner. We ate, drank and chatted about the week just gone and the week ahead, and I filled Mum and Dad in on the new song and how I'd written it. Then I told them about my Bucket List and some of my goals for next year.

After a lovely evening of catching up with the parents, they dropped me home at 8.30pm. When I got home, I sat at the piano and started to play.

*"When the day comes and you find the one,*

*there's a feeling that can't be denied.*

*It's a feeling that you want to feel,*

*every day for the rest of your life.*

*And when the time's right,*

*You see it in their eyes*

*and you know you have all that you need.*

*And those magic moments, become magic days*

*and from days they turn to magic years.*

*So when you dance with me tonight,*

*I want everybody in the room to see,*

*that I'm the girl for you and you're the man for me,*

*and if our lives should end,*

*I want you to know that I could live a million lives,*

*and I'd still choose you as mine.*

*Some people spend their lives,*

*searching for what they believe is worthwhile.*

*But I know I've found that with you.*

*And no one can compare*

*because what we have is rare.*

*I know we make it that way, in all that we do.*

*So when you dance with me tonight,*

*I want everybody in the room to see,*

*that I'm the man for you and you're the girl for me,*

*and if our lives should end,*

*I want you to know that I could live a million lives*

*and I'd still choose you as mine.*

*So when you dance with me tonight,*

*I want everybody in the room to see,*

*that I'm the one for you and you're the one for me.*

*And if our lives should end,*

*I want you to know that I could live a million lives,*

*and I'd still choose you as mine.*

*So dance with me through life."*

I sat for a while and reflected on the past week. I was so grateful to be in a better place mentally before I returned to work, and a little excited about work with my new outlook. I sat on the sofa and read a little more of my book, but soon enough I began to feel sleepy so I made my way to bed. As I lay there, I thought about all the things that had happened in the last two weeks, how amazing it was, just how much life can change in a short time. I drifted off.

"I like the song, Shelly. Are you going to get a guy to sing it with you?" Jake was sitting in 'his' chair, with a smile on his face.

"Em, yes, probably. I think it would suit it better. Thanks."

"No problem. Good to see you still have it and that you're thinking about making it a more regular part of your life."

"That Bucket List is such a good idea, Jake. I felt great after doing that today. I really can see the benefit of having one. I am actually excited about it now!"

"I told you the worst that can happen is you would feel better," Jake laughed. "Do you feel better?"

"God, yes! I feel better than I have ever felt. I feel really grateful, Jake. I mean not just to you but in general. Do you know what I mean?"

"Yes, Shell. And, you should hold onto that feeling. It's a good thing."

"I will," I promised him. "So, what are we covering today?"

"I think we should discuss your list in a little more detail," Jake answered. "We should also look at what you've accomplished in your life so far."

"I haven't accomplished much, so far, Jake," I said, feeling kind of sorry for myself.

163

"Really, Shelly?"

"I should have gone to Music College instead of doing business. I should have stayed writing my own songs instead of doing covers for all these years. I should have got into fitness earlier in life, or at least got some kind of physical hobby."

"Keep going," he said. I'd hit my stride.

"I should have done more travelling. I should have left my job ages ago and found a better one..." I paused.

"Is that it?"

"Em, ya I think so?"

"Okay, then: you have *way* too many 'should haves' in your life. When you spoke at my funeral, you mentioned that I would never have wanted a load of 'I shoulda's' at the end of my days, right?"

"Yes, Jake. You're right." I knew where this was going.

"Well, why would you, Shell? Let's look at all the things you just said. Is there anything I should have done that you can't do now?"

I thought about the question. "Well, I suppose not. Although, I don't know about going back to college to do music."

"Think of Tiffany J. Your favourite singer. Do you remember when we spoke about Jessica's friend last week?"

"Yes. What about her?"

"Well, I remember when we were all getting promotions, or moving jobs, or starting to buy houses and all that grown up stuff. I recall Tiffany going back to college to study music. I also recall, after that, she did a creative writing class. That girl was always working on herself;

164

teaching herself guitar, piano, getting to grips with the music business, going to gigs on her own to get inspiration and ideas. She didn't give up because of her age. She didn't give in because it didn't work out with the first band, or the second or the third. Do you see where I am going with this?"

"I do Jake, I didn't realise. I like her even more now."

"Yeah Shell, because it inspires you and gives you hope. 'I should have done this and I should have done that' won't get you results. It will give you regrets. Don't have regrets, Shell. There's no reason you can't do it too. The Bucket List is the best. It imprints in your mind, and that's the first step. You take the action of writing down what you want. We don't call the list 'I should have done list'; that's depressing. You said it yourself: it's more fun and it feels good to write down the things you want to do. So, let's take a look at your 'I should haves.'"

"Okay Jake, good idea."

"You said, "I should have gone to Music College instead of doing business.' So, what's stopping you? Would you like that?"

"Well, I would like to improve my musical ability."

"So, how do you do that?"

"Study Music I suppose!"

"Is there anything stopping you returning to college to study music?"

"I'm thirty-one Jake," I said with an exasperated air, "and it costs money to go to college."

"Come on, Shell! Be more solution orientated and not so problem focused. You could go back as a mature student and you could get a grant."

"True, I suppose."

"Yes, it's true. Oh yes, 'I should have stayed writing my own songs instead of doing covers for all these years?' Seriously? You just wrote a song in two hours! The years of being in a band doing covers is the only thing that kept you involved in music! Why not think of that as your practice period for performing and being inspired? *Now* you can focus on the songwriting."

"I will, Jake!" I said determinedly. "It's one of my goals now."

"That's what I mean, Shell! It's never too late! Well, unless you're in my position!" he laughed as his own little joke.

"And how about 'I should have got into fitness earlier in life, or at least got some kind of physical hobby'? Did you not just join a gym? Have you not just started going for regular walks?"

"Well yes, but..."

"No buts, Shell! You are doing it now and all the talk in the world about what you haven't done up to now won't change the fact that you didn't. So, now that you are applying action, leave it go! It's done."

I couldn't argue. He made some good points.

"And you mentioned travelling. Isn't that one we could all say? It's a big world, Shelly, but you can only see more when you move more. Plan holidays! You listed lots of places you want to visit, so take one, decide when you're going to go and let that bit of action propel you forward."

"I am. I'm going to go to Canada to visit Cara."

"Super! There you go! Make the decision and go for it. And finally, here's the best one: 'I should have left my job ages ago and found a better one.' Is it that bad?"

"Well, it's not the best job in the world Jake."

"I know that Shell, but if you can't love it, try to bring love to it and see how that goes, first."

"I don't know if I can, Jake. They're very negative! It's not exactly the most positive environment in the world now, is it?"

"Shelly, you can go around blaming everyone and everything for your lack of happiness in your work, but only you can fix it. Henry Ford said 'Whether you think you can, or you think you can't, you are right.' I think tomorrow you should, pardon the pun, start a new list. This list is to be 101 things that make you happy."

I rolled my eyes. "Another list?"

"Wasn't the last one fun? Didn't you say you could see the benefit of it and that you enjoyed it?"

"Yes, but I'm working tomorrow and I have the gym before work and then I have to meet the wedding couple. I won't have time."

"Ah, the most precious thing in the world: time. Make the time! Use your lunch break. Besides, I'm telling you this because I know it will alter your state and help you to feel good. Tomorrow you'll need it more than you have so far. The worst that can happen is it will make you feel better."

Jake smiled that charming smile of his and gave me a little salute.

"Until tomorrow, Shell."

I opened my eyes to the sound of my alarm going off. I don't know why I even bothered setting an alarm anymore at that point. It was 6 am and I had to be at The Gym at 6.45am, then be at work for 9 am. This was the first time I had been up so early before work and I was using it as a practice run. I would have to learn to be organised and schedule time at the gym. Ivan had advised me that I should be doing three sessions per week and breaking them up to work three different muscle groups. He had also explained that each group should be given adequate recovery time. Lots to think about.

I washed my face, brushed my teeth, got dressed and applied just enough makeup to make me look fresh. I didn't want to look like I was going clubbing. When I got to The Gym, I noticed that the lights were on. It was only 6.30am, but I decided to head in any way.

As I walked in, I heard a man's voice singing. I peeked my head into the gym only to see Ivan walking around doing a quick inspection and singing away to himself.

"Don't give up the day job," I said.

Ivan quickly stopped, turned toward where I was standing and laughed, "Well, seeing as you're a professional songwriter, I'll take that on board."

169

I had to laugh. "No offence," I assured him.

"Oh, none was taken. I'll restrict my singing to the shower from now on, but just for that you'll have an extra tough training session this morning."

"Don't worry I think I can handle it."

"You're pretty confident!"

"Always"

"I like that!" he said with a smile. "Very attractive quality in a woman, you know? I think that all most girls need to be attractive is confidence and a smile."

"That's a nice way of putting it," I teased. "Are these woman naked, then? Wearing nothing but a smile?"

Ivan gave that big amazing grin that had become one of those things I found most attractive about him. "I have a feeling I won't win with you this morning, so I'm not even going to try," he said, admitting defeat.

"Shall we get going?"

"We shall."

Ivan guided me through a tough session, as promised, and as I finished the last exercise I couldn't help but feel as if he was checking me out. I really wanted to ask him out. My mind was racing, and I couldn't figure out what to do.

"Small world, isn't it?" Ivan finally interrupts my train of thought.

"Sorry, I don't follow."

"The whole wedding thing, and you writing a song for it, and for one of my best friends. It's a coincidence."

170

"Or synchronicity," I responded, as I started to think about it myself. Ivan looked at me with a confused expression on his face. And then out of nowhere, I blurted out "what are you doing Wednesday night?" Ivan smiled.

"I don't know. What had you in mind?"

"A surprise," I told him. He grinned again. "I'll meet you in the car park downstairs at seven o'clock. Wear warm clothes. Don't be late."

I tried to walk out of the gym as casually as possible even though my legs were a little wobbly after the workout. I was totally shocked by what had happened. When I entered the changing room, I sat on the bench and took a deep breath to compose myself. It really hadn't been so difficult! I felt so relieved. I took a shower and left as quickly as possible before I had to face him again.

As I sat in the car, I thought about the whole incident. It seemed to happen so easily and it felt right; him singing his heart out when I arrived, the way the conversation flowed effortlessly...I'd known it was the right time to ask him out. That was two off my list already.

"Go me!" I shouted to myself as I drove off.

When I arrived at the hospital, I felt a slight dip in my energy. I remembered what Jake had advised me the night before: "You have to go in here and work with these people so change the way you deal with it and see it with fresh eyes."

I started to have a chat with myself as I sat there, listing the pros and cons of going in with a new attitude and psyching myself up to be the best darn Shelly I could be before I started to get the feeling

171

someone was watching. I looked around, and there was one of the
hospital security guards staring at me from the car parked next to mine. I
smiled and give a little wave. He stepped out of his car and closed his
door. He was still looking at me, and I started to laugh. I got out of my car
too.

"Sorry about that, I was giving myself a pep talk" I admitted.

"I figured as much!" he chuckled. "Hey, I was sorry to hear
about your friend Jake. Fierce nice fella."

"Wow, I think he knew everybody," I joked but I was slightly
shocked at this random man knowing Jake. "Or maybe everybody knew
him?"

"The latter, I think!"

"What's your name?"

"Jim." He put out his hand to shake mine.

"I'm Shelly."

"I know! Your mum is Liz?"

"Yes. That's my mama."

"Lovely lady too."

"That she is. Well, it was nice to meet you Jim; I'm heading this
way." I pointed behind me.

"Nice to meet you too, Shelly," said Jim, as we went our
separate ways.

When I arrived in the office, I was surprised to be greeted with
a bunch of flowers at my desk from my colleagues. They all made a point
of being extra nice and sympathetic. I felt slightly overwhelmed. I sat

172

down in my chair and took a deep breath. I felt genuinely lost for words. "Wow, guys! Thanks for everything but, really, I'm fine. There's no need to make a fuss!"

Fiona, who I'd never really liked, started to speak. "Poor Shelly! Rob said you were taking it really hard and might be in denial. Don't worry; apparently, that's quite normal."

I looked at Fiona, shocked. I started to feel myself getting angry.

"*Rob* said? What do you mean Rob said?" I snapped. "What does Rob know and what's he doing talking to you about me anyway?"

"Oh, I am sorry Shelly. I didn't want to upset you. It's just Rob was Jake's friend too and we are seeing each other so it came up."

I felt my blood start to boil, but luckily one of the other girls, Nora, interrupted with an offer of coffee.

"No thanks Nora," I replied. "I'm good. I think I just might head to the cafeteria."

I got up from my desk and charged across to the cafeteria like a bull. I was so mad. I couldn't believe that Rob didn't tell me. I couldn't believe this had happened to me today after I'd been in such a good mood all morning and after everything else had gone so well. "For God's sake, this is not fair," I thought to myself. As the words rolled through my mind, I started to hear my internal chatter as if for the first time ever. I stopped in my tracks and changed direction as if being guided by another force.

173

I walked towards the maternity ward to find my mother. By the time I reached the ward, I had calmed down a little. Merry little Dee was there, sitting at the reception desk.

"Hi Dee, is my Mum around please?"

"Hey Shelly, how are you love?"

"Oh, you know Dee, so, so." As soon as I spoke, it felt all wrong again. I started to become really aware that this was the way I used to feel all the time. The drama; the anger; the reacting. Eventually, I realised, for the first time in my life, there was a simple way to know how good you are feeling and that's to experience the opposite, and that was it for me.

"Shelly, are you alright pet?" Mum appeared from down the corridor.

"Mum, I am so sorry. I just didn't know where to go." I started to feel the tears welling up in my eyes. My mother knew better than anyone that I was not one for making a scene.

"Come this way with me, Hun." She guided me into an empty room.

"Sit down there sweetheart. Tell me what happened?"

"Oh Mum," I started crying. "I think I just forgot Jake was dead." I could barely get the words out. "It didn't really hit me till I arrived back here this morning and everyone made a big fuss about it. They were all drama and 'sure God love ya'. It felt wrong. And then Fiona, I mean of all people, Fiona! Well, she told me she was seeing Rob and he was talking to her about me. She said that he said I am in denial! I was just so

174

shocked. What's he doing with her? He knows we never got on. I mean, how long are they seeing each other? I know they were together when I met him last week and he never told me! And, to make it worse, he wanted to know if we were definitely over."

I swiftly moved from sadness to anger. "The cheek of him! I just...I just feel so angry at it all."

My mother looked at me with an ocean of sympathy in her eyes.

"That's a big load of stuff you had thrown at you right there," she said as she smoothed the hair out of my eyes. "I can understand why you would be angry but remember anger only hurts you – not the other person or people."

I took a deep breath.

"And to be honest, Shelly, it's probably a good thing you had a bit of an outburst. We were beginning to think you were a walking time bomb. It's normal to feel sad and angry over Jake's death and it's just as normal to release it and talk about it."

"I know Mum. I know. You're right. That sounds just like something Jake would say, too." I dried my eyes and looked up at her. "Thanks. I feel much better. In fact, I didn't even know where I was going. After everything happened in the office, I knew I had to get out of there..."

"I'm always here when you need me," Mum said. "But we'd both better get back to work. Do you want to call home this evening?"

"I have to meet the couple about the song after work but if I am not too late, I will. Thanks again." Mum hugged me.

175

"No problem pet, that's what Mums are for."

She smiled as she left the room and returned to work. I gathered myself, grabbed a cup of coffee in the cafeteria and walk back to the office. I sat at my desk and decided to start that list Jake spoke about. 101 Things That Make Me Happy. "Well, this can only make me feel better, so now is as good a time as any to start," I told myself as I took an A4 sheet from the desk and started to write.

No.1 Singing

No.2 Dancing

No.3 Funny movies

No.4 Eating ice-cream

No.5 Playing piano

No.6 Writing songs

No.7 Watching rugby matches for the hot men

No.8 Listening to Spanish Guitar

No.9 Going to gigs

No.10 Family Dinners

No.11 Playing with Samhain

No.12 Drinking wine

No.13 Going out with the girls

No.14 Christmas

No.15 Seeing an old couple holding hands

No.16 Waking up at 7 am and realising it's a Saturday and you have a day off

No.17 Finding money on the ground when there's nobody else around who could own it

No.18 Fresh bed clothes and PJ's

No.19 Sunshine

No.20 Watching a dog chase its tail

I started to get into a flow and I could feel my mood lifting, but a voice interrupted.

"Shelly, are you busy?"

I looked up from the page. It was my supervisor, Margaret.

"Hello, Margaret. No, not at all! What can I do for you?"

"I just wanted to see if you were okay."

"I'm fine, Margaret. Thanks for asking."

"That's good to hear Michelle. We missed you around the place last week and it just seems to get a bit messy without you. When you get a chance, would you mind starting a search for these charts in the archive, please? I know if anyone can find them it's you."

Margaret handed me a list of names.

"Sure thing, Margaret," I said. "No problem."

"Oh, and Shelly, if there's anything I can do, just let me know okay?"

"I will Margaret. Thanks again."

I placed my list in the desk drawer and grabbed the one Margaret gave me. But just before I headed to the archives, a thought occurred to me, "Oh crap! I forgot to organise the date for Wednesday." I quickly sat back down, searched online for the number for the night time

177

kayak place and keyed the number into my mobile. I called as soon as I got back to the office.

"Hello, Atlantic Sea Kayaking. Vicky speaking."

"Hi, Vicky. I am calling to enquire about your nighttime kayak trips. I was wondering if you have a trip this Wednesday night and if you have availability please?"

There were places available, and Vicky and I chatted for a little while. She told me what we'd need to bring, how long it would take to get there, how long the trip would last, and lots of other little details I wouldn't have thought of. I paid in advance using my card, and hung up, excited about my date with Ivan and relieved that I was able to get the booking.

I spent most of my morning in the back offices searching for the files Margaret had requested. 1 pm came and it was off to the cafeteria to get some lunch before I returned to my desk. I decided to work a little more on my list of things that made me happy. After lunch, I returned to the back office to search for the rest of the files and managed to spend most of the day avoiding the rest of my colleagues. As soon as 5 pm arrived, I was out of there.

On the drive to meet the bride and groom-to-be, I played the CD recording of my song and sang along over and over until I arrived at Tracey and Aaron's house. It was a very posh area; private estate with only five other houses. As I pulled into their drive, I saw Tracey and Aaron in the front room of the house. They spotted my car as I drove up and arrived at the front door to greet me.

"Come in, come in," said Tracey as she guided me in through a beautiful hallway. It had large cream floor tiles with a gold speck and the staircase swept around in a spiral from the centre of the hallway, leading all the way to the top floor, where directly overhead a stained glass window allowed light to pour in and reflect on the floor tiles. The living room was just as beautiful. I sat down in a comfortable armchair.

"Do you want a cup of tea or coffee, Shelly?" Aaron asked.

I asked for a coffee. While Aaron was bustling around the kitchen, Tracey turned to me with a big smile.

"So Shelly, I am so excited to hear the song! You were super quick at doing it. I mean, we weren't even sure we could make it a reality. But I knew deep down in my gut when I met you that you'd go a great job."

I felt flattered.

"Wow, thanks, Tracey. You really thought that?"

"Yes, I did. Especially, considering the whole sequence of events. I mean we thought of the idea last Monday, and between my Mum mentioning it to Mary at choir practice and Mary suggesting it to you; then you agreeing and being available, it was magic."

"I suppose you're right! It's synchronicity." I gave her a big smile. I felt really comfortable in her company and found her easy to like.

Aaron returned to the room with coffee for me and for Tracey.

"So...can we listen to it now?" he asked.

"Yes!" I said. "Of course!"

179

I handed Aaron the CD which he placed in the stereo. We all sat and listened to the song. I watched Tracey and Aaron for their reactions. I could see that Tracey was liking it. A big smile appeared on her face as she listened to the chorus. Aaron wasn't so easy to read but then he grabbed Tracy's hand and smiled at her.

"So what do ye think?"

"Oh my God Shelly! I love it," Tracey blurted out, then she turned to Aaron. "Do you like it, babe?"

"Yeah! I really like it! It's great Shelly, and you have some voice too."

"It's perfect Shelly. It's perfect," Tracey added.

"Great. I am pleased you like it. There's just one thing I was thinking."

"Yes?" Aaron sat forward, giving me his full attention.

"Well. I think it would be nice to have a male voice too; like a duet. What do you think?"

"Super idea, Shelly," Tracey agreed. "Oh! Your brother could do it, Aaron, couldn't he?"

"Good idea. Do you mind that, Shelly, or did you have someone else in mind?"

"No, that's great. It's a very basic musical piece and if your brother can play the guitar and I play the piano, we can both sing. It will sound fuller and easier to dance to as well. All we need is to have a rehearsal together. Can you guys arrange that?"

"Of course!" came the reply in unison. "When suits you Shell?" Aaron asked. "If I pass your number to Fionn, he could call you to arrange to practice. Would that be easier?"

"Perfect, that's a wrap." I must admit I was quite pleased with the outcome.

"Well, down to business Shelly. What's the cost of all this?"

"I almost forgot!" I said, truthfully. I'd just been enjoying their company. "Well, I was thinking about it and I decided for my two hours writing plus another hour for performing, it will cost €300 for my time. The song, however, is yours. Call it a wedding gift but, only, on the condition that I am known as the writer."

"Seriously, Shell?" Tracey looked at Aaron and back to me with a shocked expression.

"Shelly, whether we pay you for the song or not, you would be known as the writer. But, don't you think that it's worth a bit more to you? I have no problem paying well for something worth it. And, to be honest, having our own song at our wedding and for the rest of our lives, that's worth it to me. Are you sure you don't want to think about this a little more?"

"Thanks, guys but that's my decision. I will, however, take you up on the dress offer and I will attend the wedding. Other than that, just pass on my number to anyone you know who wants a song written."

"Done!" Aaron quickly replied.

I left the house and as I sat into the car, Aaron appeared.

"Shelly, here," he said as he handed me an envelope. "Your payment cheque is in there and a business card for Tracey's friends dress shop. Just call her, it's all arranged. Your wedding invitation is there too. You won't get in without it!"

"Thanks, Aaron! See you Saturday."

I drove home feeling very pleased with myself. It had been a productive day.

I decided to visit the family on my way. I had dinner with Mum and Dad and told them about my day before I headed home to bed. I felt exhausted after all the drama and the 'networking,' so I went straight to bed and fell fast asleep.

"Go on, Shelly! Ms Boom-Boom! I'm *very* impressed. Talk about taking action; you nearly put me to shame."

"Thanks, Jake. It wasn't all that hard, to be honest. If I was to think about it, it felt like I was guided, as to what to do this morning. All day, actually."

"That's exactly what happened, Shelly. You *were* guided."

"I knew it! It was you, wasn't it?"

"God no, Shell!" Jake said, surprised. "This here is my work. What goes on during your days is all you."

"So who or what guided me?"

Jake looked at me with a very serious expression. I could tell he had a lot to say, and I paid close attention.

"Everything you ever do in your life, every decision you ever make, or have made, or will make has two possible paths. You choose

182

Path B with your head; that's the path you choose with your thoughts, logic, analysis and experience. But Path A...well, that's what you choose with your gut. That's instinct.

"The problem comes when you don't know which path to choose. That can really stall you and stress you out, with all the negative things that involves. Even from my own point of view, I think I knew this long before I really understood it. I mean, I could understand what I was being told, but then my head got involved and went to war with my gut. I only really got used to knowing my gut by ignoring all the noise in my head. By relaxing. With practice, though, the answer always came clearly. Once I figured that out, I never doubted it. Does any of that that make sense?"

I told him that I thought it did, but when he asked me for an example from my own life, except for what had happened earlier that day, I couldn't give him an answer.

"Let's take today as an example, then," he said. "This morning, what made you ask Ivan out? Smooth, by the way. Very slick. Nicely done."

"Well, firstly, he was singing. Just belting it out. It was nice to see that side of him and to know he can be a bit goofy. He's not, like, some sort of full-time demigod all the time." That got a laugh out of Jake. "Anyway, that was a sign that put me at ease. Then, the conversation was easy. It just flowed and I felt confident. So, when the opportunity arose, I just grabbed it!"

"There you go, Shell! That confidence was your gut. It was guiding you and that's why it was easy. It's that feeling of confidence in the real sense of the word. I mean, it's not ego; it's our natural state of confidence like when we were kids and we were full of confidence and joy. If you watch a child playing or doing anything, really, you'll notice a big difference: They don't over-analyse situations. They don't over-think. They don't care what people are going to think if they start dancing in the middle of a shopping centre or if they decide to sing a song while they're out for dinner! They live in the moment. They have no idea what it's like to feel paranoid!

"However, adults feel paranoid all the time! That gives us a reason to stress out, which gives us *another* reason to stress, and then we get worried, and then we worry about being worried before we start to overthink everything, which gives us more to think, worry and stress about. It's really the hard road."

He really had a point. Everything he said struck a chord with me, especially when he pointed out that people get stressed about getting stressed. It's like we never even give ourselves a chance!

"Even today," Jake continued, "when you were bombarded in work, you could feel yourself getting ready to explode and you left the situation and where did you go?"

"To my Mum," I said. "I was actually going to the cafeteria but something changed my mind."

"Yes, Shell. You followed your instinct. And then what happened?"

184

"Well. Mum helped me to calm down and feel better."

"Exactly! Do you think that going to the cafeteria would have had the same effect?"

"No. It would have probably made me worse. Especially, if I ran into somebody from the office."

Jake nodded, sagely.

"Can you think of a time in your life where know you were following your instincts?"

I had to think for a while.

"I suppose the time I ended it with Rob. I couldn't tell you why, but something didn't feel right and I felt it was time to end it. I didn't even really understand it myself at the time but, after today, maybe it was my gut guiding me. It was telling me he wasn't the one for me."

"Yes, Shell! Good example. But, it becomes even clearer further on down the road, be it a week, month or even years later, doesn't it? Things work out for the better. In all our lives, we have experiences where our gut guides us and we never think about it and things work out perfectly. Then, there are times when things don't work out and we often hear or say, 'I had a gut feeling about that. I should have listened to it.'"

"That sounds an awful lot like yet another 'I should have'" I said.

"I suppose it is, Shell. But, are you understanding any of this? Does it make sense?"

"Yes, I am." This was making more sense to me than I'd expected, especially after the day I'd just had. "Overthinking is usually not the best way, and even if we're not aware of it, our first instinct is often the best solution."

"Well said, Shell. Has the student become the master? Very eloquent!"

"Why, thank you kindly, Mr Lawlor" I replied, with exaggerated politeness.

Jake gave me an encouraging grin.

"I was really impressed with how you decided to charge them. It was very fair and very kind."

"Yeah, I know," I admitted. "I couldn't decide and when I arrived at their home, I knew that they had money but it didn't matter. I like them as people and I feel privileged to be a part of their wedding and their whole life, to be honest. That song is theirs now."

"It was a lovely gift," he said. "I have no doubt, it's only the beginning of your songwriting career. I bet they'll pass your number on to loads of people willing to pay for their very own wedding song."

"True. I wouldn't mind earning a quick grand to book a flight to Canada for next year. That'd be another goal in motion!"

"I think you're starting to like these lists, Shelly. Did you enjoy writing the list of things that make you happy?"

"It actually saved me today from being dragged into the drama and negativity at work! It did help me feel happier. In fact, I'm beginning to think that writing, in general, is quite enjoyable."

"Do you think that? Or is that your gut telling you?" Jake joked.

"Ha! Ha! Funny man."

"Always. It's time to say goodbye again."

"Already?"

"Until tomorrow. Remember: listen to your gut and you won't go far wrong."

"Okay, Jake. Bye."

I stared out my window at the dark sky. There were still a few stars visible. I thought about Rob and Fiona. I really hadn't seen that one coming, I wasn't surprised. I decided that I wasn't going to let it get to me anymore. At work, I was going to just relax and follow my gut. It was only 6.30am, so with plenty of time I got up, showered and went for breakfast before work.

As I was getting ready, I spotted the envelope Aaron had given me. Inside was the business card for Tracey's friend's dress boutique along with the wedding invitation.

*Aaron Miller & Tracey Higgins*

Would like to invite

*Michelle Morrissey*

To share in their special wedding day

On November 8<sup>th,</sup> 2013

Wedding ceremony @ 1pm in

*Thorn Hill Church*

Followed by reception

*At Lake View Hotel – R.S.V.P*

It was only then that I looked at the cheque Aaron had written, and I swiftly did a double take. Aaron had made it out for €3,000, not €300. I was stunned. Attached to the cheque was a little note that read:

*Dear Shelly,*

*I want to start by saying it's been a pleasure to work with you and I think it was a very thoughtful and kind gesture you made with the song.*

*I know the cheque is for a bit more than agreed. This may not be the value you put on your work, but it is the value I put on it. I calculated based on the joy on Tracey's face when she heard it. When a job is done well, ahead of time, to the highest standard, it ought to be rewarded.*

*Thank you for the kind gift that we will have for our lifetime. Looking forward to seeing you Saturday to share in the celebrations.*

*Kind regards,*

*Aaron*

I was blown away by it all, especially the cheque. It was far more than I had ever considered asking for. In fact, it was the most money I had ever made for any kind of work. I jumped with excitement as I suddenly realised that I could book my flight to Canada and even have some money to spend once I got there! I felt like an excited teenager and I gave in to the urge to jump around my room. Jake was right: following my gut had been exactly the right thing to do.

I grabbed my handbag and headed for breakfast. I made it to the Coffee Dock by half seven, with plenty of time to have breakfast and

189

still beat the heavy traffic to work. I sat by the window as always and ordered.

"I hope that's black coffee," said a deep, familiar voice.

I looked up, into the smiling face of the beautiful Ivan. He sat down across from me with a takeaway cup in his hand. "Are you not coming to see me this morning?"

"Aww," I mocked; "did you miss me?"

He smiled and said, "Yes." He looked as if he wanted to say something else, but couldn't decide if he should.

"Go on," I prodded him.

"Are you really taking me on a date tomorrow night?"

"I don't know Ivan. Am I?"

"Well, I hope so, now, because I have rejected at least ten other offers since yesterday. So, don't tell me I disappointed them for nothing!"

I deliberately ignored him. I was enjoying being a tease.

"Why aren't you at work, anyway?"

"Oh yeah, change the subject! I just popped out for a coffee, that's all. So? What are we doing?"

"It's a surprise, just meet me like we arranged."

"A surprise...I see. I suppose you want my number, then?"

"No," I said with a shrug. "Not really, thanks!"

"That's a bit harsh!" He told me. "Are you sure we are going on a date? Because I am starting to feel like this is a bit of a wind-up!"

"Just be there," I said demurely.

He gave me a long, hard look with a smile at the corners of his mouth, then got up to leave.

"I know you like me so don't play so hard to get. Enjoy your breakfast!"

We smiled at each other for a moment before he turned and left. He strode out the door of the coffee shop and I watched as he walked across the car park with a coffee in one hand and his phone in the other. He disappeared around the corner and I turned back to my breakfast. Suddenly, my phone beeped. I had a new text.

*I already have your number. Was going to text you later. I guess we were meant to meet this morn. Have an awesome day :-) X*

I was ready to explode with joy and excitement. I had butterflies. After breakfast, I drove to work and parked the car in the hospital car park as normal. I walked into the office building and spotted Fiona on my way.

"Hey, Michelle. How are you?"

"Great, thanks" I replied. Time to bury the hatchet. "And you?"

"Oh, good, I suppose." She suddenly appeared very uncomfortable. "Listen," she said. "I'm sorry about yesterday. It wasn't a good time to drop that information on you. I'm sorry."

I looked at her for a moment and took a deep breath.

"Fiona, no need to apologise. Rob and I are over a long time and we were never really serious anyway. So, don't feel bad. In fact, I think you two are very well suited and I wish you both all the best. Plus,

191

my best friend just died and I need to deal with that more than with anyone else's drama. I'm sure you understand."

"Of course. Thanks, Michelle."

"No problem. I'm heading to the cafeteria to grab a coffee. Do you want one?"

"No, thanks, Michelle," she replied with a surprised tone.

"Fiona, my name is Shelly. That's what my friends call me, ok? See you in the office."

As we walked in opposite directions, I felt really good about what just happened. It was like the day I met Rob and, instead of getting mad, I stayed cool and relaxed. The words just flowed out of my mouth and I think the results were good, compared to the way I used to behave and the reactions I used to get. As Jake always said, 'treat others as you would like to be treated.' I knew it was going to be a good day. I could feel it in my bones.

I grabbed my coffee and returned to my desk. I decided to add a few more bits to the list of things that made me happy:

No.21 Going out for dinner with friends or family

No.22 Santa Claus: The Movie

No.23 Playing Jenga

No.24 Walking and kicking leaves in Autumn

No.25 Playing in the snow

No.26 Travelling

No.27 Trying new food

No.28 Reading magazines

No.29 Watching 'Sex in the City'

No.30 Celebrating my birthday

No.31 Going to the cinema

No.32 Flying

No.33 Playing on a trampoline

I stopped writing for a minute as I had an urge to check my phone. I'd put it on silent after Ivan's text earlier so I could concentrate on getting to work without driving into a wall from sheer delight There were two messages and one missed call. The missed call was from an unknown number. When I checked my messages, there was one from Ivan and one from the unknown number.

*Can I at least have a clue?*

I laughed at the message as I thought of what to write in response. A minute passed, and then another as I figured out what I wanted to write. Eventually, I played it safe:

*A special activity in a peaceful environment.*

After I responded to Ivan, I moved on to the message from the unknown number.

*Hi, Shelly. Fionn here. My brother Aaron gave me your number to contact you about rehearsal. Tried to call but I assume you're working. I'm around any evening, can call to you if you like. Have a copy of the song and have been playing it on the guitar. Let me know what suits for a practice. Looking forward to it.*

I had to think for a moment as to when would be a good time to rehearse? Mindful of everything Jake had been teaching me, I decided not to procrastinate. Why not that night?

*Hi, Fionn. I am free this evening around 7 if that works. Would be good to do it as soon as possible and if we need to do one more before Saturday then we will know tonight. I have a keyboard and guitar at home if you want to pop over to my house. My address is 39 Camden Court, Castletown. It's the first house on your left at the back of the estate. Look forward to meeting you :-) Shelly*

After hitting send, I grabbed the list from the day before and headed to the back office to find the last few missing files. I searched through row after row, looking for the ones Margaret was missing. Just before lunch, Fiona walked in.

"Shelly, are you in here?" she shouted as she stepped over the boxes on the floor.

"Back here!" I answered.

"Oh, there you are!" she said as she tried to avoid the boxes on the floor. "I was just wondering if you wanted anything from the Coffee Dock. Theresa and I are going to place an order and collect it. Just for a change from the cafeteria."

"Actually, that'd be great!" I stepped down from a little ladder and moved toward Fiona. "Can I have a chicken, salad and pesto wrap, please? Toasted."

"No problem." Fiona wrote down my order on a piece of paper.

"Do you need the cash?" I asked as I wiped a stray bit of dust from my forehead.

"No, it's ok," said Fiona. "You can sort me out when we get back."

"Great. Thanks."

As she stepped over the boxes on her way out, I realised how much I appreciated the gesture, even if it was unexpected. I grabbed the last two files, put the boxes back in order and headed back to the front office. I put all the files together and brought them to Margaret's office.

The girls returned with lunch and we all sat around eating, chatting and drinking tea. I couldn't help but feel a little better about my job and I begin to question what it was I used to complain about in the first place. Maybe the job, the work and the people were never the problems. I sat there and looked around the office at everyone for what seemed like the first time. I saw it all differently and I realised that, just like Jake had explained, it was not the situation or people you had to change but yourself. I got up and walked across the room to Fiona and handed her some money.

"Thanks again," I said, with as big a smile as I could muster.

"No problem!" she replied with an equally big grin. "It was a nice change, wasn't it?"

"Definitely! I love their food. We should make it a Tuesday tradition."

"That's a great idea," said Fiona. "There's only so much canteen food we can take."

I returned to my desk and got stuck into the pile of work waiting for me. The afternoon went by quickly. By the time I looked at my phone, it was nearly five o'clock and there were a few more messages waiting for me. One was from Fionn to confirm our rehearsal tonight, and one was from Eve asking what was I up to for the night. The last message was from Ivan.

*I'm intrigued, by our mystery date and by you. See you tomorrow.*

I packed up my work for the day and gathered my belongings, said goodbye to everyone in the office and headed home. As I hopped into the car, I set my phone to hands-free to call Eve.

"Howdy! What's up?" Eve roared down the line.

"I'm on the way home from work to do a rehearsal for the wedding I'm singing at on Saturday," I told her, "then, I must get myself organised for my date tomorrow night." That almost shocked her into silence, but being Eve, that didn't last long.

"What? A date? With who?"

"Ivan!"

"Ivan?! Oh! My! God! How did that happen?"

"I asked him out, that's how!"

"You did what?!" Eve was clearly astonished at this revelation, and she started laughing down the phone. "I'm calling over tonight," she informed me. "I'm not taking no for an answer. We need to catch up."

I knew she meant it, and that she'd just wait on my doorstep if I told her I wasn't going to be there.

196

"I should be done with rehearsals around eight or nine, so I'll buzz you after and you can pop over for all the scandal." We chatted about a few other bits and pieces, and I hung up just as I arrived home. I got inside, put on the heating and quickly changed into more comfortable clothes. After a quick bite to eat, I put my living room into rehearsal space mode, and at 7 pm on the button, the doorbell rang. I opened the door to be greeted by a young man with a guitar.

He was extremely personable, and I invited him in. His face lit up with a grin as he walked into the living room/rehearsal area. He inspected my old keyboard with an impressed look and strummed my guitar approvingly. While we were getting set up, we chatted about our experiences on the music scene. I was a fan of 'Aces and Stars', his group.

"That's pretty impressive," I said. "You guys have a great reputation."

"Yeah, they're a great bunch and it's a fun job. I love music; it's a pleasure to be able to do one thing I love and make enough to pay for me to go to college and do another thing I love."

"I hear you are studying to be a doctor?"

"Yup! I've heard a bit about you too; your voice is very nice, and the song is lovely."

I felt appropriately flattered.

"That's very nice of you to say," I smiled. Then, it was time to get down to business. I played the song from the top and Fionn played along, getting a feel for it. He'd been practising since the night before so

197

he was pretty confident when it came to the guitar line. We played the song through, and then we played it a second time splitting the verses up between us. I sang the first chorus, we shared the second verse, Fionn sang the second chorus and we both sing the chorus again together to finish. A few goes later, the results were outstanding.

"Nailed it, kid!" Fionn exclaimed, putting his hands up for a high five.

I laughed as I gave him a high five. It had been much easier than I expected.

"That's what it's like when professionals work together!" Fionn joked. We played the song one more time and decided that we ought to give it another run-through on Friday to keep it fresh in our minds. When we finished, I looked at the clock. It was just 7.40pm.

"That's a good day's work Fionn," I said as I switched off my keyboard. "Well done. I must say, I really like your voice; very pleasing to the ear and easy to sing with."

"Thanks, Shell," Fionn said with a slightly self-conscious smile. "Well, I better get going!" He stifled a yawn as I walked him to the front door. "I need an early night. I'm still exhausted after the weekend."

"Oh yeah, the stag! How did you get on?"

"It was epic. It was the best stag ever! Some of us did a hill climb, and at the top of the mountain, they had bikes waiting for us and we got to cycle down. What a rush! Then we hit the pub, the club, and the bed, and we were up the next morning to jump out of a plane. Awesome!

Definitely, need to catch up on some sleep tonight." He yawned again as he headed out the door and I wished him a safe journey home.

As soon as Fionn was gone, I texted Eve and told her to call over. She stormed in the door about fifteen minutes later. I could hear her running up the stairs to my bedroom. She burst in and jumped on me, pushing me over onto the bed. She was never one for a quiet entrance.

"I can't believe you asked him out!" she shouted. "How did you do it? Fill me in!"

I laughed at her enthusiasm as I tried to push her off of me. "Eve! Get off me, you crazy person, and I'll tell you!"

Eventually, she relented and sat at the end of the bed. I started laying out clothes for the next day as I filled her in about how I asked Ivan out, and about the weird coincidence of him being friends with Aaron and Tracey, and all about the cheque for €3,000 and Aaron's lovely note. Then, I told her about the work drama with Rob and Fiona before finishing up with the rehearsal with Fionn.

"Is he hot?" Eve asked.

"Yes, actually. He's very good-looking, but he's only 22 years old, Eve!"

"Yeah, but he is a musician and he's studying to be a doctor. I mean, seriously, Shelly. He could make me better and sing to me at the same time."

We chatted for another while about my big date with Ivan, then Eve headed home and I went to bed and thought about all the times over the day where I'd followed my gut instincts and when I'd followed my head, and about the wedding and Ivan and work. It felt like my mind was racing too fast to ever fall asleep, but it wasn't long before Jake arrived, so I must have fallen asleep more quickly than I expected.

"I have absolutely no idea what to expect on this date," I murmured, half to him and half to myself.

Jake put on his sports commentator voice

"Shelly Morrissey! Welcome to your 15$^{th}$ sleep! Today, we will be mostly discussing the greatest joy you can experience!"

"Okay, Jake. But can you please tell me first what the heck I'm going to do about this kayaking?"

"You're useless at playing along!" he teased. "Kayaking is loads of fun. You're going to love it. They'll kit you out, though, and it'll be chilly, so one word of warning: wear warm clothes for under your extra-large wetsuit!"

I hadn't even considered that. My heart sank. "A wetsuit?! Oh no! Not the most attractive outfit for a first date."

Jake raised one eyebrow. "Seriously, Shell? He's seen you all sweaty in a tracksuit; I don't think he is going to care. Besides, guys don't think like that and you'll both have too much to distract you from thinking about it. Being out at sea at night in a kayak is one of the coolest things I ever did. It's amazing. I can't wait for you to see the sea lighting up!"

"Does that really happen?" I asked. I'd heard about it, but I always thought it was just a myth,

"It totally does," he said. "You run your paddle gently along the top of the water, and the plankton starts to glow. It's beautiful, and it only happens in a few parts of the world."

"Wow, Jake. That sounds amazing and beautiful."

"It is! He'll be impressed when you're able to tell him all about it, so make sure you look up all the details."

I was aware of a little half-smile on my face as I thought about glowing water and the impressed look Ivan would give me when I explained it.

"But that's enough of that for now," Jake said. "There really is something I want to talk about that isn't Ivan or plankton. Do you remember how you used to mock me for doing random nice things?"

"Oh ya! You had some sort of a stint going around buying homeless people food and carrying old people's shopping. But, they were all very good things to do Jake. You know I was only joking."

"I know, but what I don't think you know is that that doing those things gave me the greatest gift of all. I don't know how to explain it, but there's no greater gift you can give yourself than giving to others. It's a buzz like no other."

"Okay, Gandhi! I believe you."

"Gandhi said 'be the change you want to see in the world.' I really believed in that. So I put out there what I wanted back. I donated platelets for nearly a year. Every month, I went into the blood bank and gave a donation. I loved going in there giving my donation. I was so grateful to be able to do it."

201

I smiled at the memory of what a really deep-down good person Jake had always been. It was no wonder I'd loved him so much.

"I got more joy out of doing that then you could imagine," he continued. "I swear the hospital staff in the blood bank thought I was a bit strange because I was probably the happiest person donating."

"What was it like?" I asked him.

"You get hooked up to a machine that takes blood out of your arm, runs it through, separates and removes the platelets and then returns the blood back to you through the same arm."

I winced. "That sounds...ouch."

"A little bit," he admitted. "I had to stop a few months back after I had a bad turn and got sick in the middle of the donation."

"What? Really?"

"Yeah, it happened twice on two different occasions but the first time I just got weak and felt faint. The second time I actually threw up. The doctor told me not to donate platelets anymore for a while. I was so disappointed! I could still donate blood, but I had to just take a break for a few months."

"I don't think I'd be into that," I mused.

"It's not that bad, Shell. Besides, you have a tattoo! If you can do that, trust me, you can give blood."

"Fair point," I conceded. "I'll put it on my list."

"Good! It'll be easy for you: You work in the hospital so you can pop over anytime and do it. I know you'll feel good doing it, Shell, and if not, then just don't do it again. But please give it a go, at least once."

"Yes!" I said determinedly. "My mind's made up; I'll do it."

"Another thing I loved to do that I never told anybody about was to randomly pay for people's stuff."

"You did what? What do you mean 'randomly pay for people's stuff'?"

"How many times have you seen somebody on the street begging?" Jake asked me. "Have you ever noticed that sometimes they have a sign that says 'I am hungry'?"

"I see people begging all the time Jake," I answered. "There are so many it's hard to know who is genuine or not." Jake sat down on the bed and looked me in the eye with an expression of sincerity on his face.

"If you think like that all the time, you just might miss the opportunity to help a person truly in need," he said. "You might miss an opportunity to touch someone's life."

He had a point, I knew, but I wasn't prepared to let mine go.

"Yeah, but I might also be avoiding giving to someone who doesn't need at all."

"That's the thing with money," Jake said with a mild scowl. "I don't believe in giving money. I always gave food to those who were hungry, clothes to those who were cold and time to those who were lonely. I never saw the sense in throwing money at people. If you see a person with a sign that says 'hungry,' go to the nearest shop and buy them some food. It's the best feeling ever to help another person,

203

especially if they are hungry or cold. Nobody wants to be hungry or cold, Shell. Food and warmth are basic human needs."

"You're right," I admitted. "It's as simple as feeding someone who doesn't have food."

Jake nodded.

"Yes, it's that simple. One time my friend Martin was out shopping with his girlfriend, and they were behind this young guy in the queue. Martin watched as the guy went through his pockets to try to come up with enough money for his groceries. Long story short, he didn't have enough so he left the loaf of bread and took what he could afford. When Martin got to the checkout, he grabbed the loaf of bread and asked the assistant to put it in with his groceries. He walked over to the young guy and gave it to him before returning to the till to pay."

"Ah, that's so nice, Jake. It's so like Martin to do something like that, though, isn't it? What did the guy say?"

"He barely said anything, Martin said. He was probably shocked, maybe embarrassed, or maybe even insulted. Martin didn't make a big deal of it. He just said, 'I did it because I wanted to and you never know. That guy might return the favour someday and do a kind act for someone else.' It's better to do a good thing instead of wishing you had."

Jake could see I was thinking long and hard about what he was saying, and he let the silence hang in the air for a little while longer before he continued.

"It doesn't have to be a big thing, Shell. It can be something as simple as giving someone your time if they're lonely, or volunteering at the hospital to read to sick kids or helping someone with their shopping..." Jake started to laugh. I asked him what was so funny.

"I just had a memory of this old lady. A few months back, I was on my way home from The Gym, walking down Low River Walk, and I came across this old lady taking a rest on her way up the hill. She was sitting on a wall catching her breath. I stopped and offered to help her with her shopping. She handed me the smaller of her bags and I asked did she want me to take the bigger one also? She wasn't too keen on giving me the other bag...I think she had her purse in it. In any event, she wasn't too sure of me. I walked with her for what felt like a half an hour and, you know me, I was all chat. She barely spoke two words. She just nodded and agreed. Eventually, we got to Stanton Road and she reached out for the other bag. I handed it to her and that was that. I don't even know where she lived! I just turned around and walked away. I really think she thought I was going to rob her or try to find out where her house was and was she alone. Anyway, I don't know but it did make me realise that it's so rare that people do nice things for no particular reason that people have become so suspicious now when you do. It's kind of sad."

He had another point. It really was sad, but the mental image of the look on the old lady's face was pretty funny.

"That was really nice of you, Jake. I wouldn't know what to say or do. I'd probably overthink the whole thing."

"Most people do," he agreed. "They think about doing something good, but instead of just doing it, they get worried about the reaction. Then they tell themselves they don't have time. Eventually, before they know it, they've talked themselves out of it. That's why people have lost faith in one another. Our gut instinct is to help, and our brains take that away."

"I know," I said. "I can see that, now."

"Another good one is to buy a tea or coffee for whoever's behind you in the queue at a coffee shop."

"You mean a total stranger in the queue?"

"Yeah, that's the best part! You look back at a random someone and say it to the cashier. In the Coffee Dock, they have regular customers so the staff usually know what people are having."

"That sounds a kind of a fun idea. I might just do that one!"

"One time Sam paid for this guy's coffee," Jake reminisced, "and as we were leaving the coffee shop he was staring at her trying to figure out whether or not he knew her, or maybe wondering if she fancied him. She said she kept seeing him on the street for ages afterwards and he always had the same confused look. It was pretty entertaining."

"It's like the film...what was it called?"

"*Pay It Forward!* Exactly! Whatever inspires you and feels good, go for it. The worst that can happen is you feel better! You feel better for doing it than if you didn't. I used to try every day to find a good deed to do. I got a real buzz from it...I even got a date out of it once. In fact, I gave my last ever bit of change to a guy who was short money for his bus ticket."

That was bittersweet but definitely more sweet than bitter. Jake saw that I was in danger of becoming sentimental, so he made sure to stay as positive and enthusiastic as only he knew how.

"When it comes to giving, Shell, it shouldn't be restricted to strangers. I reckon it should always be a priority to give to family and friends."

"As in presents from when you're on holiday or socks at Christmas?"

He chuckled at my little joke.

"I'd be thinking more about time. I think that arranging dinner parties or outings or random dates to spend time together and give the other person or people your time and attention can be overlooked. Making someone feel special or supported in their own lives is a wonderful thing to do...why wouldn't you want to do that for your family and friends all the time? If one of your friends is going through a tough time, take them out for some fun or cook them dinner and just give them your time. Tell them about how wonderful they are! If things are going well, make a big deal of it and celebrate with them. To me, that's what being a friend means."

He was right. Looking back on all the times he'd done that for me, I felt grateful and inspired.

"I'm going to host a party for the girls," I announced.

"Good!" Jake exclaimed. "Great! Super idea!"

207

"I want it to be themed, I think...although that means I have to think of a theme!"

"That part's easy!" said Jake. "There was that party that Martin had for his housewarming where we all had to pretend to be living our dream lives. If you were in a job and you wanted a promotion, you spoke as if you had it, if you were waiting on the keys to a house you acted as if you had the house, or if you really wanted to be in a relationship you spoke as if you were in the perfect relationship. Were you there?"

"No, but I heard about it...probably from you! It was good?"

"It was hilarious. One of the best parties I ever went to. Everyone was happy."

I was trying to remember why I hadn't gone.

"Why wasn't I there?" I asked.

"Maybe you were playing a gig?" Jake suggested.

"Probably! I thought Martin and Jen had ignored me!"

"God, no Shell! Martin wouldn't ignore anyone. Jen had to take over the organising as Martin was asking too many people! We actually had to point out to him that it was in his house, not the White House and there probably wouldn't be enough room."

"True," I said. "They're both lovely. I must pop over to them soon. I didn't really get to chat to them much at your funeral. Jesus, there's another thing I bet nobody's ever said before!" We both burst out laughing.

"That's a perfect place to leave it for tonight, Shell," he said. "Another sleep is ending. Enjoy the date tomorrow night, and most importantly have fun. Remember the plankton!"

"I will Jake! Thanks."

I jumped out of bed and got ready to head to the gym. It was a wet morning and I hoped that it would dry up before I brought Ivan on our date. I couldn't stop thinking about him as I drove through the rain. I parked as close to the front door as I could so I wouldn't get too wet running in.

Diane was her usual bubbly self at reception, and we nattered briefly about the weather and the forecast before I went into the changing rooms, where I took my work clothes out of my bag and hung them up, grabbed a small towel and my water and made my way back out.

Mark was waiting for me, with a big smile plastered across his face. He'd be training me, not Ivan. I felt a little pang of disappointment.

"Ready to get down to it?" he asked, and Diane laughed when she saw the apprehension on my face.

"Don't worry, Michelle," she teased. "He's a softy really."

Mark laughed, "Yeah, right! Follow me for a session to remember, Shelly." I followed him into the gym. Did he know that I'd asked Ivan out? I decided to play the innocent.

"All on your own this morning, then?" I asked.

"Just till eight, then Nicky and Ivan are in. Until then, we have the place to ourselves. So, it's legs today! We are going to start with some calf raises. Then squats followed by lunges, some RDL's and, lastly, quad extensions. Okay?"

I understood at least some of what he was talking about. It sounded intimidating.

"Okay, I suppose. But I have to be at work for nine!"

Mark looked at the clock. It was 7.30 am. He looked back at me.

"Okay, smart ass! You just earned yourself a leg press on top of that."

"You are going to torture me, aren't you?"

He responded with an exaggerated, movie-villain laugh, and clapped his hands, rubbing them together. It was time to begin.

I started with calf raises. After I finished them, he had me do 3 sets of 20 squats, followed by 3 sets of 20 lunges. I started to struggle on the last set but Mark didn't give me the opportunity to slack off. Motivation seemed to be his speciality.

That morning was my first time attempting a Roman Dead Lift. My legs wobbled and quaked, but to my surprise (and delight) I managed to do it. Last, but not least, it was quad extensions. I sat into the machine and Mark set it up. I looked at the weight. It really seemed to be a lot.

"Are you for real? I am a girl, you know, not a Terminator!"

Mark just laughed.

"Nicky would do that with one leg!" he teased. "Besides girls need to lift heavy to build muscle, and muscle burns fat. You'll appreciate the benefits, believe me. The quicker you do it, the quicker it's done."

211

"No shit," I said, still apprehensive. I didn't feel like this was something I could do quickly.

I did the first set. Then Mark dropped the weight. On the fourth rep of the second set, I felt dizzy. I felt weak. I'm sure Mark saw the colour drain from my face. I started to break into a cold sweat. I was sure I was going to get violently sick. Mark figured out something was up and went from trainer mode to comforter mode.

"It's alright Michelle. Just breathe. It's just a release of growth hormone. It will pass; just keep breathing." It was no good. In spite of Mark's soothing voice and reassurance, I bolted, barely making it to the changing rooms and into the toilet before throwing up. After a few minutes of just sitting on the floor of the toilet, I heard a girl's voice calling me.

"Shelly, are you okay in there? It's Nicky."

"Hi Nicky," I said in a weak voice. "I'm fine. Just...give me two minutes."

I gathered what remained of my strength, then slowly dragged myself up off the floor and walked out into the changing room.

Nicky smiled kindly.

"Oh, the memories. Don't worry, Shell. It's happened to me so many times."

"Don't tell me you've gotten sick training?"

"Hell yeah!" she laughed. "Loads of times! Especially after Mark. He's got a gift for it!"

Nicky sat with me for a few minutes until I felt better and had some colour back in my face.

"How do you feel?" she asked.

"I'll live," I said. I was already feeling less woozy.

"I should hope so! Don't you have a date tonight?" she winked.

I didn't know where to look.

"Don't worry Shell! I won't tell him you got sick. We can just say, you thought you were going to so you came into the bathroom, but it passed. Okay?"

"Thanks, Nicky. How do you know?"

"Ivan and I are close. When I came to work on Monday, I noticed how happy he was so I asked why he was in such good form. He couldn't wait to tell me! No-one else knows, though. Don't worry. Besides, Ivan usually never dates clients, so he'd be very private that way."

That made me feel much better about everything.

"Thanks for everything, Nicky. I'd better hop in the shower and get ready for work."

"Good idea! The shower will sort you right out. Enjoy tonight; I can't wait to hear about it."

She was right: after my shower, I felt much better. I got dressed and ready for work. It was 8.20 as I made my way out of the dressing room and into reception. Ivan was in the gym with a client, and we caught each other's eye. He smiled that radiant smile at me and I did my best to look like I hadn't just been sitting on the floor of the bathroom. "Later," I mouthed, grinning from ear to ear. He gave me a thumbs up, and that

213

alone made me feel better than anything Nicky or the post-vomit shower had.

The traffic was really heavy on the way to work. It gave me plenty of time to think, and I went over and over what Jake had said to me the night before. What better way to start my random acts of kindness than by doing something nice for my colleagues? I changed route and popped into the Coffee Dock to grab fresh scones for the other people in the office. When I arrived in, a little late, I piled the scones, cream, butter and jam on the table and told everyone to help themselves, and it was smiles all 'round; a much better way to start the day than arriving in with a scowl and grumbling at people! Teas and coffees were collected from the cafeteria, and we all sat and ate our scones and had a chat before getting down to work. It put everyone in a good mood for the day.

Seeing everyone with a smile on their face made me so pleased I'd done what I did, and I decided it was something I should make a habit of. By lunchtime, everyone in the office had come up to me and said thanks. I went out for lunch, as I wanted to lodge my cheque. It had been in my bag for days and I knew it would be safer to lodge it in the bank. Putting that much money into my account felt great, too. Once I got back to work I was kept busy for the afternoon, setting up a new filing system for the office and reorganising old files.

The day went by in a flash. Before I knew it, it was five o'clock. I grabbed my bag and coat and headed home to get ready for my date. I knew it would be dark and cold, so I didn't put too much emphasis on my clothes, but I did freshen up my makeup for the car journey. After getting

214

ready, I boiled the kettle, filled a flask of hot water, got a small carton of milk, some sugar, tea bags and coffee and put them into little tubs. I packed spoons, too, and a packet of biscuits.

I was ready for the road. After a last check in the hall mirror, and a moment of staring myself in the eye and telling myself it was going to be great, I locked up and drove to collect Ivan.

When I pulled into the car park, I could see his Jeep in the spot where it had been that morning. I wondered had he been there all day. He walked out the door, and I started to feel butterflies. I watched him walk to his Jeep and grab a bag from it. He swung it nonchalantly as he made his way to my car. The butterflies increased their speed as he opened the passenger door and sat in.

"Hey! How are we doing?"

"Great! Great! I'm doing great! Uh...and you?"

"Pretty damn good, thanks," he said. "So, where are we going?"

"I told you, it's a surprise."

"I know, but I'll be as surprised now as I would be when we get there."

"Good point," I admitted, "but I prefer to keep you wondering."

"That's fair enough," he admitted. "How far away is it?"

"About an hour."

"A whole hour to get to know each other!" he beamed. "I'll start. What made you want to ask me out?"

I laughed.

"I didn't actually ask you out, you know. I asked what you were doing on Wednesday night, and you presumed I was asking you out."

"Yeah, yeah, yeah," he mocked. "Whatever! Just admit it! I mean, it's cool. I like that you asked me out."

"Well, really I needed to fill the gap in my diary for Wednesday night," I joked.

He laughed again. "You're a gas ticket. Oh, I hear your song is awesome. Aaron was saying."

"Oh, really? That's good, I'm glad he's pleased. His brother came over to my place last night. We tried it together."

"If I didn't know what you were talking about," Ivan said exaggeratedly, "I'd be jealous."

I had to think back to what I'd just said. When I caught on, I laughed, "God Ivan, you're sick! He's like 22 years old."

"Oh, Fionn is well able for the ladies. He's been a toy-boy more than a sugar daddy. He likes older women."

"Too much information!" I giggled. "I won't be able to concentrate when I see him again if you say anymore."

"He's a good catch, don't you think? Good looking, talented, smart and rich."

"It sounds a little like you have a boy crush!" I teased. "Are you sure you don't want to go out with him yourself?"

"Well," came the answer, "if we don't work out, he can be my Plan B."

216

"Plan B distracts from Plan A, don't you know?" I said, demurely.

We both laughed and continued chatting all the way to Reen Pier. I could tell Ivan hadn't been expecting this at all.

"Okay...what the heck are we doing here?"

"We're going kayaking!" I said triumphantly. His eyes lit up.

"Cool! Nighttime kayaking! That's a surprise! I think I like it!"

"Ever done it before?" I asked.

"No, never. You?"

"No, it's my first time."

"Your first time?" Ivan asked, holding back his laughter. It took me a second to figure out what he was getting at.

"Oh my God! You have a one track mind!" I punched him playfully before we got out of the car, put on our extra layers and walked over to the group of people waiting by the kayaks. The owner, a really nice man called Jim, was going to be our guide. There were two other couples in our group. We were all given wetsuits, and we got a quick induction from Jim before he took us down to the kayaks.

"Front or back?" Ivan asked.

"Front for me, I think. You're the man. You can steer."

"Perfect. Glad you made that call," he smirked.

We took off and followed Jim. He talked about safety and guidelines for kayaking at night. It was dark and as we made our way out in the bay, quiet and still. Jim instructed everyone to take off, enjoy the space, and just keep an eye out for each other and not drift too far apart.

217

Ivan and I paddled for a little and then stopped, appreciating the tranquillity.

"It's nice, isn't it?" I said. "What do you think?"

"It's awesome!" Ivan said with delight. "How did you find out about this?"

"My buddy Jake told me about it. He went on a date here once. They loved it."

"Do you miss him, Shell? It's so soon after, still."

"I do. It's kind of surreal, you know? I suppose, in time, I will have moments where it starts to feel normal, but right now...anyway. I just want to enjoy my life. When he died I realised that I need to live for now and not waste time. Life is what happens while you are making plans, as they say."

"I really admire your attitude," he said gently. "I didn't know him well, but when he was going out with Nicky, I met him a good few times and I really liked him. I could tell he was a good guy. He just got on with everyone. That's rare."

"Yeah," I agreed. "He...he was one in a million. I'm so glad I had him in my life. He taught me so much and I'm only starting to see it now." This was getting heavy. Not ideal first date material. I decided to change the subject. "Wow, it's amazing how quiet it is out here, isn't it? I mean, we're not that far away from land, we can see the houses and places around the pier, but it just seems like another world."

"Yeah," said Ivan contentedly. "It really is lovely."

I tried to turn around to see him, but the bulky wetsuit and life jacket made it difficult. After a few attempts, I gave up. "How's the back of my head looking?" I asked instead.

"It's beautiful, Shell."

"Ah, thanks."

We heard the sound of a whistle drift across the water. Jim called everyone together and we all made our way over to a different area. He paddled along beside us and he and Ivan got chatting about seeing the world and all the places Jim had been. He was a very interesting guy and I enjoyed listening as he talked about his adventures. After a few minutes, he signalled to us all to stop paddling. As we drifted a little, I noticed a dim swirl of light at the surface of the water, like thousands of distant stars just beneath the waves.

"This is being emitted by marine life," Jim told the group. "Stay in by the bank and watch your paddles as they travel across the top of the water." It was even more beautiful than I'd imagined. I was transfixed. Ivan and I spent the rest of our time drifting through the ethereal glow, watching it ebb and flow and sparkle around the bow of the kayak and the blades of the paddles before Jim said it was time to return to the shore. We pulled our kayaks out of the water and carried them up onto the pier. Now for the really tough part; wetsuit removal.

As we started to struggle with the tight suits, I almost fell over several times, with my knees and elbows at all sorts of ridiculous angles. Ivan seemed to think it was the funniest thing he'd ever seen.

"Shelly, I know it's only our first date but I have to tell you...I'm loving the way you're getting out of that wetsuit."

I stared him right in the eye with a serious expression on my face and started to slowly pull the wetsuit down over my shoulders, doing a sexy little dance. We both started to laugh. After we thanked Jim and said goodbye to the others, we headed back to the car, cold but exhilarated. I turned to Ivan.

"So...did you enjoy it?"

"Michelle," he said sincerely, "I'm well impressed. Cold as hell, but well impressed." This was really my moment to shine.

"Well, I have a flask of hot water in the car so we can make a cuppa before we go. If you're really good you can have a biscuit, too."

He shook his head in wonder.

"Wow."

I waited for a smart comment, but none came. Ivan wasn't just looking at me anymore, he was gazing. I could feel myself starting to blush, so I dove out of the door and got busy making tea. I grabbed the flask from the boot and we sat quietly in my car, enjoying our tea and biscuits. We were facing the sea and we could still just about make out a slight glimmer from the water as the waves came in softly onto the shore. By the time we had finished our snack and warmed up a little, it was nearly 10 pm.

"Time sure does fly when you're having fun," Ivan said softly.

"I'd better get you home," I said.

220

We chatted all the way back, with no awkward silences, and it seemed like to no time had passed at all as we pulled into the car park at The Gym.

"Thank you," he said earnestly. "I really enjoyed tonight. It was awesome."

"I am glad you enjoyed it," I smiled. "It was a pretty random thing to do on a Wednesday!"

"So, I suppose it's my turn next?"

I turned to him with a cheeky grin on my face.

"Are you asking me out?"

"It'd be rude not to return the favour," he answered with a smile.

"Yes, it would," I said.

"Okay. Prepare to be blown away. When are you free?"

I honestly didn't know. I started totting up my obligations in my head.

"I have to rehearse tomorrow night..."

"I have a guy gathering for Aaron on Friday, before the wedding..." Ivan said, running through his own mental checklist. "And speaking of the wedding...are you bringing a date?"

"No. I am flying solo. Well, I'll be hanging with Mary, Jake's mum. Are you bringing a date?"

"Yeah, I am, actually." I wasn't expecting to feel as let down as I did, and I did my best to hide my disappointment.

"Oh...right! Who?"

"You."

My relief was palpable, and I could feel myself start to grin from ear to ear. I didn't care.

"Will you save a dance for me?" he asked.

"I might," I teased, "if you're lucky."

Ivan leant in close and whispered in my ear, "I already am."

He moved his hand around the back of my head, ran his fingers gently through my hair and pulled me in close. We kissed. When it ended, I whispered back "Yeah, you are."

He looked at me and smiled. I felt lost in his eyes.

"I'll see you in The Gym?" he said.

"Yes. Friday? I mean, if you're working on Friday? Are you working on Friday? It's okay if you're not, I mean…" I was babbling.

He leant in once more, kissed me again, got out of the car and smiled that big, bright smile.

"I'll see you on Friday."

I felt weak as he closed the car door, and as I watched him walk away. I was so happy I could have burst. As soon as he got into his Jeep, I started my engine and drove away.

All that fresh air and excitement had me exhausted, and I couldn't wait to talk to Jake about everything. I got into bed thinking about everything that had happened since Ivan closed the door of The Gym behind him and walked to my car. My mind kept drifting to that amazing kiss at the end of the night. I felt like a teenager again. It wasn't long before I was fast asleep, and Jake arrived.

"Do you like this boy? Is he respectable? Does he have land?" he said, teasing me.

"Yes, I do like him, Jake. I really do. What do you think of him?"

"Well, that really doesn't matter, now, does it?"

"I suppose it doesn't really matter what anyone thinks except me," I said, "but I'd like to know what you think."

"What I think is completely irrelevant!" he insisted.

"Because you know I'll go and do what I want anyway?" I asked.

"No, because I'm dead!"

I looked at him, stunned. He broke out laughing.

"Ah come on, I was bound to use that line a few times. It's not something you get to say too often, you know? Lighten up! Ok, I'm sorry. Tell me more about Prince Charming. Or should I start to call him Ivan the Great?"

"I don't think so, Jake," I said. I was actually feeling a little annoyed at his attitude towards his own demise and him mocking Ivan.

"Ah come on, Shell. Ok, he's a really nice guy. Don't you think I would have warned you if he wasn't? So, yes. I like him. I approve."

"Thanks," I said icily. "So why didn't you warn me about Rob, then?"

"What about Rob?"

"Well, he's dating Fiona from work and he was seeing her when he propositioned me last week."

223

"Michelle, you and Rob broke up months ago. He was still into you and probably wanted to be sure there was no hope of you getting back together. Rob's a great guy and that hasn't changed, but he's perfectly entitled to date whoever he wants. Besides, you ended it. Move on, let go and be happy for him that he is trying to get over you. Cut the guy some slack. And what's wrong with Fiona? I thought you two were getting on now?"

"Yes, we are, and there's nothing wrong with her. I'm actually beginning to think she might be nice. Lately, I hear myself and I'm surprised at how ridiculous I sound sometimes when I complain or react to things."

"You're just starting to wake up and become more aware, Shell. And I'm sorry about my 'I'm dead' crack. I know it upset you."

"It's ok," I told him. "It's just strange, you know? You're here with me, but I know you're gone, too. And I know we won't even have this, soon. I don't like thinking about it. Anyway...did I imagine it, or did you say we were going to talk about having fun?"

"Yes Shell, I did. It's quite like last night when we talked about giving."

"I did that this morning, actually. It set a good tone for the day and made work much more pleasant. In fact, I think work is much better nowadays in general."

"Do you think work has gotten better or do you think that maybe *you've* changed, and work just appears better?"

224

"Yes," I admitted. "You're right. That's what's really going on. Regardless, it's a good thing."

"It is, isn't it?" I could tell he was relieved that I didn't seem to be angry at him anymore. "And it's not that hard to do, is it?"

"All it took was some consideration and about five minutes of my time," I agreed.

"Having fun and just being happy sounds simple," Jake continued, "but it seems to have become the hardest thing to do for most people. They seem to be so busy working, planning, stressing and worrying that there's no time to have fun and just be happy. I was at a funeral recently...not my own..." he gave me a cheeky grin and I shot back an exaggerated scowl; "It was my friend Christopher's mother, and her cousin happened to be the priest. He was a great storyteller and a great philosopher, as priests go. He told a story about a fisherman from Kerry."

"Is there anything I can do that will make you not tell me that story?" I said, feigning boredom.

"Not a thing!" Jake replied with a grin. "Once upon a time, and all that! So anyway, this fisherman went out to sea every day and caught enough fish to support his family. Every day, he went out and caught the same amount of fish; no more and no less. Early one morning before he set off, as he lay on the dock by his boat, a businessman was passing by on his way to work. The businessman stopped and said 'what are you doing there?'

'I'm taking it easy,' replied the fisherman.

'People like you have this country the way it is' said the businessman, getting annoyed. 'It would be more in your line to get out and do a day's work.'

'And then what?' asked the fisherman.

'And then you can make money and support your family.'

'And then what?' asked the fisherman.

'Then you could work harder and make more money!' said the businessman.

'And then what?' asked the fisherman.

'Then you could buy a bigger boat.'

'And then what?' asked the fisherman, again.

'Then you could hire a few locals and create employment and help the economy!' said the businessman, warming to his theme.

'And then what?' asked the fisherman.

The businessman started to get annoyed.

'When you've worked hard and built a business, you might have a good business to pass to your kids.'

'And then what?' asked the fisherman.

The businessman was getting really angry now, so he raised his voice and shouted, 'and then one day you can stop working and take it easy.'

The fisherman looked at him and said 'you mean, the way I'm taking it easy right now?'"

I laughed. So did Jake.

"That's a good story. I like that," I said. "Fair play to the priest."

"Father Eamon. He's a cool guy. And best funeral I was ever at...up until my own."

"Jake! It's still not funny!"

"Ah but it is!" he insisted. "Life is to be lived the way you want to live it, and it's there to be lived right now. If you want to be happy, be happy *now*. If you want more fun, have more fun *now*. People do it backwards most of the time. 'If I had the perfect job, the perfect partner, the perfect figure, perfect health, more money, more stuff, a bigger house, a better car...' the list goes on and on. We think that we'll be happy if we can just get more stuff, or change one more thing about ourselves. That's not how it works. In order to stay happy, you have to be able to feel happy in the first place!

"I learned that a long time ago. We all make the mistake of searching for someone or something to make us happy when we should be happy ourselves. Then we can look for someone to share our happiness."

That really struck a chord with me. I think I'd just been starting to realise it over the last few days and it was good to hear Jake put it into words.

"Shelly, life is too short to do anything else. All joking aside, I have the right to say that."

"You do," I agreed, "but there are still times in life when bad things happen and it's a little harder to be happy. It's difficult to be positive all the time."

"I know," he said. "You're right. Those times are times when you can experience contrast. That's as important as being happy and having fun. But, at the same time, we need to remember that when we're not experiencing a challenge, it's the perfect time to experience joy. I think I learned that from Martin. He was the only other friend I had who had a hard childhood. His dad was an alcoholic too, but he died younger than mine. His mother learned to live from her experiences and she raised her kids to be happy every day, to make up for the days that they hadn't been happy. It's kind of strange, and sad, that the happiest person I knew in my life had the saddest childhood."

It was sad, but it also gave me a lot of hope and perspective to hear. I knew Martin pretty well through Jake, and he really was a happy, jolly, friendly, considerate good guy. It was no surprise that Jake and he got on so well, though I hadn't known how similar their childhoods were before now. I asked Jake if he thought having led similar lives, with similar mothers, had a lot to do with their shared perspective.

"Yes, I do Shell. I think happiness can be a choice, and it's a choice we both made. We're all born happy; just look at any baby or young child. Take Samhain for example." Even the mention of my little nephew made me smile. "He's the perfect example of happiness. He smiles and laughs all the time, completely naturally, with no effort. He is just bursting to smile and laugh all the time. I think that kind of sums things up, you know?"

"It totally does," I said. "It's like...when you hear the sound of laughter, and you look for where it's coming from like we are drawn to it. It's instinctive."

"Exactly! Our natural state is happiness, but then adults come along and stunt it with 'Oh don't do that' and 'don't do this' and 'don't go there' and 'don't play with that' and 'stop doing that' and 'don't break that' and 'what are you doing that for?' And if you ask questions, you get 'don't be cheeky' or 'don't you ask questions.' Before we know it, we're all acting just like the adults we once swore we wouldn't grow up to be."

"True Jake, so true. So where does that leave us, Dr Fun?"

"If it's not fun try to find the fun in it, and if you can't find the fun in it, don't do it!" I laughed again.

"Sounds good, Jake."

"I think people just need to relax more and try not to take things too seriously," he said. "That's a good start. And try to spend time with people who are fun!"

"I have an idea about that already, actually."

"Go on," he encouraged.

"I'm going to invite the girls around on Friday night for drinks, and it's going to be a *hell* of a lot of fun!'"

"Ah the party, yes, of course!" he said. "That'll definitely be a good laugh. Who are you going to invite?"

"Well, Claire and Fran, Eve, Sam, my Mum, your Mum, Dee, Sarah, Fiona and Orla from work and Nicky and Diane from The Gym.

Oh, and I might call Martin's Jen and Brian's Alice. I haven't seen them in ages."

"Good on you, Shell! Nice mix of people."

"Ya, it'll be fun, and it'll keep me occupied before the wedding."

"Oh yeah, speaking of which; are you all set for it?"

"I think so. I have another rehearsal tomorrow with Fionn but he's really good so it's easy. It just flows."

"Yeah, I was listening in. It definitely makes it more full with the male voice and the guitar."

"I'm glad you think so. I wasn't too sure but I plan on recording it tomorrow night and getting the girls to have a listen on Friday, maybe."

"Good idea. It's nice to get other feedback before the performance and boost the confidence."

"Yeah, I'm looking forward to it. The wedding, that is. It should be a good day."

"And a perfect opportunity for you to practice having more fun."

"I will, once the song is over!"

"No! You have to enjoy everything. Remember; the more fun you have, the better you become at having fun."

"I suppose that's true. Okay, I'll have fun. I'll have fun rehearsing, I'll have fun picking a dress, and I'll have fun booking myself in to get my hair, nails and makeup done. All fun, all the time. Sound good?" Jake chuckled.

"I think you've got it."

"Loud and clear!" I said.

"Time to say goodbye" Jake sang, in a terrible Andrea Bocelli imitation. I cringed, and then laughed, and then he was gone.

On Thursday morning and I woke with a strange feeling in my legs. I attempted to get out of the bed and nearly fell over.

"Oh my God!" I thought to myself, swearing under my breath. "He broke my legs! This can't possibly be normal!" I tried to walk across the bedroom, then struggled to get myself ready for work. I was lucky I had gotten up early, everything was taking far too long. Even driving was painful. I vowed never to allow Mark to train me again. The man was clearly a sadist.

When I got to work I attempted to walk across the car park into the office. Jim the security guard saw me and knew something was up.

"Shelly? Do you want me to get you a wheelchair?"

"Everyone's a wiseass," I thought to myself.

"No thanks, Jim. I'm fine," I said through gritted teeth. "I just went too hard at it in the gym yesterday."

"No kidding," he said, with a look of genuine pity on his face. "Well, take it easy!"

"No choice…" I admitted as I limped past him.

After what seemed like half the morning spent inching my way through the corridors, I finally managed to get to my desk. Before I could start work, I had to call the dress bar and sort out an appointment to get a dress for the wedding.

"Irene's Dress Bar, Irene speaking" came the answer.

"Good morning. My name is Michelle Morrissey; I got your number from Tracey Higgins?"

"Oh yes, you're the composer?"

'Composer.' I liked that.

"Yes. That's me."

"Okay...the wedding is this Saturday...you're cutting it tight! What size are you, Michelle?"

"I'm a 10, I suppose."

She still had a few sizes tens left, and we discussed some details about what I was looking for and what she could do for me. She warned me I'd have to try to make it over as soon as possible or risk not having anything at all. I made an appointment for lunchtime, hung up the phone and started to work on a pile of files I had to organise. That took me pretty much up to lunchtime. As I made it to the end of the last one, I checked my mobile. There was a message from Ivan:

*Hope you are good this morning. Just wanted to say thanks again for a super evening. I have a great idea for the next date. Guess! :-)*

In spite of the pile of paperwork and the ridiculous pain in my legs, I could feel my face splitting into a huge grin. I had to resist the urge to start giggling.

233

*Hey, Mr! So...my legs are broken. Seriously. I think Mark is trying to kill me. But anyway, you're very welcome. And my guess is next date will be a surprise? :-)*

I hit send and tried to stand up.

"Ouch! Damn it! Ah, crap! Christ!"

I made my way across the office, shuffling slowly and swearing enthusiastically with each step. Tom looked up from his computer in the corner with a mixture of concern and amusement on his face.

"What, in the name of God, has you walking like that?" he asked, slowly shaking his head in bafflement.

"The stupid trainer at the gym, that's what. That crazy man is what has me walking like this. We went at it far too hard."

He guffawed.

"Jesus, Michelle that sounds bad! Are there female trainers there too?"

I stopped and thought about what I'd just said, and I could do nothing but roll my eyes and blush slightly as the whole office started to laugh.

I transfixed him with what I hoped was an icy stare.

"Tom, you have a one-track mind."

"I know. It's great, isn't it? Do you want me to grab you a wheelchair?"

I had a feeling wheelchairs were going to be a running gag for the day.

"Oh," I said, with exaggerated sweetness, "that's so *kind* and *thoughtful* of you, but no thanks. The walk will loosen me out. It's good to see everyone in top smart-ass form, though."

"I don't know about that Shelly," pitched in Fiona. "The loosening out, that is. Rob had one of his lads' train me last week and I swear I was crippled for ages. He kept saying 'walking will loosen it out.' Keep working your legs, it will loosen them out, blah, blah, blah! Nothing worked. There was no loosening. I swear, I thought I was going to be like that forever."

"Great. So there's no hope for me?" She laughed, and I couldn't help but grin too.

"Actually Shell, a bath..."

".....in Epsom salts," I finished her sentence. "I know. I'll definitely have to do that tonight. And I'd better get a move on or I'll have an accident."

I hobbled my way down the corridor to the toilets and hobbled back again. After the stress and strain of that simple task, I arranged the work I had to get done after lunch, made my way very, very slowly to my car and drove to my dress appointment. I arrived at Irene's Dress Bar, drove around the back and parked. There were steps up to the door. I looked at them in disbelief. I couldn't catch a break.

"Oh come on, give me a break!" I appealed to nobody in particular. After I made my way up all eleven steps, I tried to open the door but it was locked. I knocked on the door. A slim dark-haired woman opened it.

"Hello, Michelle. How are you, dear? I'm Irene. Come on in."

"Hi Irene," I said. "Thanks for seeing me on your lunch."

"No problem dear. I just hope you like one of the dresses I have left!"

"I am sure I will, Irene. I'm not all that fussy."

"Oh but I am, my dear! I can't allow anyone go out in one of my dresses if it doesn't suit them. It makes me look bad."

I started to laugh at the funny joke and then realised she wasn't kidding. She made tutting noise, then presented me with a pile of dresses, all covered in plastic

"Take these over to the other side of the partition and try them on," she ordered. "Only call me if you think a dress has potential. Okay, dear?" I obligingly gathered the pile of clothes and shuffled over to where she'd shown me.

I tried on the first dress. I didn't like it. Then the second, Oh, no! No, no, no. The third was terrible. The fourth was awful. But, the minute I saw the fifth dress, a red fitted cocktail dress with a low scoop back, a scoop front and decorative gold bracelets across the back, I just fell in love with it. It fitted like a glove. I had honestly never felt a dress fit so comfortably, or look so good. I started to feel really excited.

"Irene!" I called. "I have it. I found the one!"

"Marvellous!" she declared dramatically. "Let me see it!"

I walked out from behind the partition and stood up as straight as my aching legs would allow.

236

"Oh, my word! That's the dress for you alright, my dear. That's the one. That's a dress that could take all eyes off the bride. That," she said, arching her eyebrows over her trendy glasses, "is what I call a danger dress. A dress that makes a girl look so good, they could take another woman's man. You're practically a weapon."

I decided that this woman was very strange, but that I liked her a lot. She was like a character from a play, and she fussed and clucked as she walked in circles around me, appraising the dress from every angle.

"Yes, yes, yes, oh my *goodness* yes, yes absolutely, yes." She seemed to be going through some sort of mental checklist. Both the dress and I met with unqualified approval.

"Yes, you are highly dangerous. There simply isn't another dress in the world which would look that good on you. Pop it off, dear," she ordered. "I'll rewrap it for you so it doesn't get dirty."

"Thanks so much," I said, as she set about giving me a list of directives about when to return it, how to hang it...even how to fold it. Again, she looked over the rim of her glasses with a deadly serious expressing.

"This is extremely vital, Michelle. You must make no attempt whatsoever to wash this dress. I have my own dry cleaners and they will collect all the hired dresses from the weekend on Monday evening. They, and only they, are authorised to wash my dresses. Yes?"

I felt like perhaps I ought to salute.

"No problem, Irene, and thanks so much."

"You are most, most welcome," she said with a look of prim satisfaction on her face at a job well done. "I hope your man appreciates how remarkable you look. If not, he is a Philistine. Enjoy the wedding."

And that was that. Irene said not another word and opened the door for me. That was my cue to leave. I walked slowly down the steps, still feeling the pain from yesterday's workout with every step. By time I got back to work, I barely had time to grab a coffee and a wrap. I ate at my desk, before returning to work mode. Thinking of how Ivan would react when he saw me in the danger dress made me happy. I decided to follow through with my party plans there and then, and send out e-mails and texts to invite the girls around for drinks and fun the following night.

The rest of the afternoon passed so quickly, as had the week, that by 5 pm I was surprised with how much work I'd gotten done. While I was on holiday my workload had piled up a little, but with my first week back nearly done I felt really happy with my progress. In fact, I was starting to enjoy work and my work environment much more than I had before.

On the drive home, I noticed my legs were much looser. That made me feel even better about everything. As I drove, I thought of all the things I needed to get done for the busy weekend. I needed to stop at the shop and get some finger food and snacks for the girls and more Epsom salts for me. I also had to clean my house, get organised for Saturday and do a practice run of the song again before the following night's rehearsal. And I needed to check whether Eve had a pair of gold shoes I could borrow which could go with the dress.

238

Once I'd made my mental list, I realised I hadn't heard any more from Ivan. Maybe he was just busy, or maybe he was playing hard to get. 'Or maybe,' said a little voice deep inside, 'he doesn't like you as much as you thought he did and…' And then, just as I started to overthink everything, my phone rang and it was him. I lit up like a Christmas tree and had to remember to sound like a calm, cool, collected woman as I answered the phone.

"Hey," I said, as nonchalantly as I could. "How are you?"

"I'm great!" he replied. "How are the legs?"

"Actually, they're much better, thanks! I just bought Epsom salts so I'm going to have a nice relaxing bath before bed. That should sort everything out."

"Sounds good. Need any help with that?"

I giggled at his cheeky comment, like a teenage girl.

"Thanks for the kind offer but I've managed to have baths all by myself since I was six, so I have a good 25 years of experience under my belt. I'm very proud of myself because of that! I'll manage."

"I'm sure you will," he said, "but it's way more fun when someone else helps."

"Maybe next time."

"I'll hold you to that"

"I bet you will!"

I smiled at how easy and entertaining it was talking to him, and we spent what felt like ages just talking about our respective days, who we'd met, what we'd done, the funny and interesting things we'd seen or heard, and a million and one little details I'm not sure I'd even have noticed before I met him. I told him all about my party plans and he told me all about last-minute wedding prep with Aaron.

Just as it occurred to me that this meant I probably wouldn't even see him until the wedding itself, he asked me whether I was going to show up for training in the morning. In the middle of everything else, and in spite of the painful reminder every time I moved my legs, I'd almost forgotten.

"If you let that nutcase Mark anywhere near me, I swear to God you'll never see me again!" I warned him.

He laughed.

"In that case, I'd better take charge or your training personally. I swear, I'll take it easy on you. So...will I see you in the morning, then?"

"You'd better take it easy!" I said. "I have to perform at this wedding and the last thing I need is to be in pain." I could hear the smile in his voice when he answered me.

"I promise, I will be very, very gentle," he said, seductively. I laughed and told him to knock it off, though I think he could tell from my tone that I didn't want him to knock it off at all. We chatted for another minute or two before he had to go and meet a client for a session.

After hanging up, I sat in the car and thought of how amazingly fast things can work out sometimes. Seeing how quickly a different attitude can help to effect a change made me feel a greater understanding of all that Jake had been teaching me. It felt good. If he hadn't come back to help me, I realised, my life couldn't possibly have become so good so fast. When I got home I made some dinner, then I blasted music and started cleaning the house from top to bottom. I actually really enjoyed it, and by the time I was finished it was about nearly half past eight.

While I waited for the water to heat up for my bath, I went over the song a few more times, playing around with the harmonies and starting to feel really comfortable and confident. After an hour had passed, I made my way upstairs to have my bath before bed. While I was in my bedroom packing for the gym the next morning, my phone went off. A text message from Eve.

*Hey, Shellybelly! I've a pair of divine gold saddles and a pair of nude ones too. I'll give them to Mum and u can get them off her in work. Am away in Galway 4 d wknd so won't make the party sorry :-( but have fun!!! Good luck on Saturday and enjoy. Can't wait to hear all about it and about d date.*

*Love u XOXO*

I replied, finished packing and hopped into the bath. After a good soak and reading a few more chapters of my book, I felt very relaxed and very tired. I got out of the bath, dried off and dressed for bed. I was asleep as soon as my head hit the pillow.

"*Galileo fell in love as a Galilean boy and he wondered what in heaven...*" Jake sang as I sat up in the bed. He serenaded me with the whole song. It was lovely. Finally, he finished and asked me how I was. I sighed with contentment.

"I am fantastic, Jake. Thanks."

241

"You're just transforming right in front of me, you know," he said with a look of genuine happiness on his face. "I am so proud of you."

"You're doing a good job," I told him. "So, what's on the agenda today?"

"Never giving up, Shell. And learning to let go."

"That sends a little bit of a mixed message, don't you think?" I said, a little confused. "Aren't they sort of the opposite of one another?"

"It depends on how you look at it Shell, and we're going to look at it from two different perspectives. Are you ready for story time?"

"Sure. I love stories!"

"Then listen closely!" he said, dramatically.

"Once upon a time...wait, have you ever heard of Colonel Sanders?" The name rang a bell, but I wasn't sure why.

"Who?"

"KFC? Glasses? Smile? Little Van Dyke beard?"

"Oh yeah, I get you. I know who you're talking about."

"He was the founder of Kentucky Fried Chicken. His story is pretty cool, actually. He retired at 60 years of age and had to live off social security, which was a pittance. So, he decided to use the only thing he had that might make him money; his fried chicken recipe. He drove all over America visiting restaurants and cooking for the restaurant owners, and he told them that if they liked his recipe he'd let them use it for a small percentage of the profit. He slept in his car and often the only food he had was the chicken he'd cooked at the demonstrations. Take a guess how many times he heard the phrase 'no, thank you'."

"100?" I said. Jake shook his head. "200?" Nope. "500?!" Jake was still shaking his head.

"1,000?!?"

"More!"

"Who hears 'no!' more than a thousand times and carries on?" I asked, exasperated.

"He heard 1,009 people say 'no' before someone eventually said 'yes,'" Jake said.

"That's...actually really impressive. In fact, I think it's amazing. I can take one or two people telling me, no, but after that, I pretty much just move on to the next thing" I told him.

"I know! And I felt the same after I heard it," he replied. "But don't jump ahead yet, keep your thoughts on hold until I tell you the next one."

"Okay Jake," I said, feeling like an eager student. "I'm all ears."

"Okay, once upon *another* time, there were two monks on a pilgrimage. One day, they came to a deep river. At the edge of the river, they come upon a young woman. She was crying because she was afraid to cross the river on her own, and she asked the two monks if they would help her. The younger monk turned his back because members of their order were forbidden to touch a woman. But the older monk picked her up and without a word and carried her right across the river. At the other bank, he put her down and continued on his journey.

"The younger monk crossed over too and walked after him, tutting and sighing. After walking all day, the older monk finally asks the younger man; 'what is the matter, brother?' The younger monk started to scold him for breaking his vows and touching a woman. He went on and on like that for quite a while, getting angrier and angrier.

"Eventually, after listening to the younger monk for far too long, the older monk said 'I only carried her across the river but you have been carrying her all day.'

"The younger monk stopped talking, and the older man could finally enjoy a minute's peace."

Jake looked at me waiting for a reaction; "So?"

"Colonel Sanders is a very inspiring guy. That's pure tenacity."

Jake agreed.

"I suppose I never really thought about life that way," I went on. "I never actually wondered what made famous or successful people famous and successful. I've never really thought about how they got there. They never give up. Well, until they are successful."

"Yes, Shelly. Very well said. And what about the monks?"

"Well...it shows that when something happens that you don't like and you can't change and which doesn't really affect you in the first place, you shouldn't carry it around. Let it go. And I can see why you told me both stories back to back; it makes sense because you need one to counter the other, sometimes. They don't cancel each other out so much as *balance* each other out. You just need to know when you ought to do one instead of the other."

I could tell Jake was impressed, whether at his teaching or my learning.

"Spot on, Shell. Simple yet effective. I used to tell those to a lot of the kids I used to train. They loved them. But who doesn't like stories, right?" I nodded in agreement.

"Everyone likes stories, Jake. You don't have to be a child to appreciate a good one."

"That's exactly it Shell. The best stories are the ones about real people having real experiences. That makes them easier to connect with. Like you said earlier, you'll never look at KFC the same again; that's because you have created a new association with it and it's positive. I never even ate KFC except for once in a blue moon...in fact, I don't think I went near the place for ten years before I died. But when I heard that story, I couldn't help but get a nice feeling about the place because of it. It's a happy ending." He was right. It wasn't a fairy tale and it wasn't some sort of parable, it was just a story about a real guy who made something of himself. I wanted to hear another.

"I don't want to use up all my stories Shell."

I cajoled him and did my best sulking face, and eventually, he relented. He thought for a moment, and then he began.

"When I was in college, my philosophy lecturer told us a story about a psychologist who was teaching stress management.

"One day, this psychologist was walking around with a glass of water in her hand. She walked into a lecture theatre, got the class's attention and held the glass up. They all presumed she was going to ask the usual question: 'is the glass half empty or half full?' but instead, she asked 'how heavy is this glass?'

245

"She got lots of answers back. Everyone wanted to have a guess. After they'd all had their say, she said 'the weight of the glass is irrelevant. Let me show you.'

"She got a girl from the class to stand up and hold the glass out in front of her. 'Do you think that glass is heavy?' she asked. 'No,' responded the girl. 'Ok' said the lecturer. She chatted away to the rest of the students while the girl held the glass straight out in front of her for a minute, and then she asked again: 'is the glass heavy?'

"The girls responded 'not really but my arm is getting tired.' 'Aha!' exclaimed the psychologist. 'Your arm is getting tired but the glass hasn't changed in weight. So, what if you held the glass there for a half hour?' The girl responded, 'I'd have a dead arm.' The class laughed. Then the psychologist asks, 'what if you held it for a week?' The girl, with her arm dropping down a little, said 'I'd be crippled!'

"'Exactly,' said the psychologist. 'The longer you hold it the heavier it seems. The stresses and worries in our lives are like that glass of water. Hold on to them for a few minutes and it's fine. Hold on to them for an hour and it begins to affect you. After a day you're in pain. After a week, you might be doing yourself some real harm. You can become crippled by them and you feel incapable of doing anything. It's important to let go and put them down as soon as you can. Don't carry them all day and all night, don't carry them for a week, or a month, or a year, or a lifetime.'"

That story, in particular, resonated with me.

"I like that one a lot. Smart lady."

246

"Yeah, I like it too," said Jake. "Your turn now. Tell me a story."

"I don't know any stories!" I protested.

"Seriously?" he asked. I nodded. "Well then, you're going to have to make your own story. Go out there and live, and someday, you'll have an amazing story to tell. And when you do, I'll be listening."

I promised him I would. I told him that I felt like a work in progress, but I was feeling optimistic about a happy ending for perhaps the first time in years.

"Speaking of endings, I'd better say goodbye now until next time."

And then Jake was gone again, and I woke up alone in my room pondering the lessons I had just been taught.

After staying in bed for quite a while, I began to associate the difficulties in my life with Jake's analogy of the glass and I started to see how, most of the time, it wasn't the actual problem that affected me: it was the way I held onto the problem and didn't look for a solution. I saw how Jake might have found that side of me difficult to be around.

I thought about all the times when Jake offered good advice and I chose not to accept it. I would just brush it off as overly positive 'motivational speech' stuff. There were even times when Jake just listened to me moan and complain, even though I knew he'd have had a lot to say. I don't think I realised until then, though, that Jake had always been trying to help me in one way or another. I'd had a bad attitude, and I chose to be that way. I didn't want to be like that anymore.

I had only four more visits from Jake left to look forward to, and I knew I'd better make the best of the time we have left. I had to make my story a good one. I rolled out of bed, got dressed and freshened up before leaving for The Gym. When I got there, Ivan was at the front desk.

"Dossing, Mr Casey?" I teased.

"Would you listen to Ms Morrissey? All smug and smart so early in the morning!" He grinned that big lovely grin and I suddenly

248

couldn't think of a single smart thing to say, so I just smiled back. "Get your ass into that gym and I'll show you what dossing is."

"I'm shaking in my boots," I said. "Back in a minute, so."

I strolled into the changing area and dropped off my bag, then returned to reception. Ivan nudged me towards the gym.

"Come on then, and I'll take it easy like you begged."

I gave him a little punch in the arm.

"Easy there, Hulk Hogan," he said, holding his arm in mock agony. "That's assault! Okay, so it's arms today…" he began to organise the equipment. "We'll start with triceps dips. Give me three 20s."

I completed the first exercise, and I was surprised to find the dips were getting easier.

"Triceps press next!" Ivan directed. When I finished those, Ivan handed me the dumbbells and I did some curls, nice and slow. Then shoulder raises with a lighter set. It wasn't easy, but I felt like I'd turned a corner because they weren't remotely as difficult as before. I was feeling cocky.

When I finished the 20 shoulder raises, I looked at Ivan smugly.

"Is that it?" He raised his eyebrows and laughed.

"No! That's just one set! We have two more to go'" He handed me lighter dumbbells, and I started again. By the time I reached the last six reps, I was struggling big time. All my smugness evaporated. Ivan smirked as he watched me grit my teeth and knit my brows.

"That's what we call muscle failure," he explained. "Pick up the 1.5 kg dumbbells and do the last 20."

I grabbed the 1.5kg dumbbells with no questions and no backchat. After I'd struggled to do the first ten, I felt like giving up.

"I can't do it," I protested. "My arms are dead!"

"Come on Shelly. You can finish these. You can do this."

He placed his hands under my arms and guided me through the last ten raises. When they were done I dropped the weights to the floor and started to rub my arms.

"Oh my God almighty that was horrible! My arms are burning!" I moaned. Ivan laughed at me.

"Don't be such a girlie," he grinned, relishing his turn to be a tease.

"I am a girl!" I shot back, "what else am I supposed to be?! Thanks, though. Ow. Ow, ow, ow." He laughed again and I gave him a mock scowl, throwing in a little pout for good measure. I struggled to raise my arm to look at my watch.

"Oh, it's eight o'clock! I'd better make a move and hit the showers or I'll be late for work."

"Cool," said Ivan. "Give me a shout before you go?"

"Okay."

I made my way to the changing rooms and hopped in for a shower, struggling to use my arms. It was particularly apt after the story about holding the glass that Jake had told me the night before. I could identify with the poor psychology student. As I flailed around uselessly, I started to come up with my own analogy. I'd used lighter and lighter weights, but by the end, there was still a lot of pain. I decided they were

250

like stresses or worries: It wasn't until I had dropped them completely that I was able to start to recover, and it wasn't about how heavy they were, but rather about how long I held onto them while repeating the same action over and over. That's what led to pain and failure...and the pain and failure were a vital part of the process of improvement and of growth. I felt quite pleased with my flash of insight.

I got dressed for work, slowly, and made my way out to reception. Ivan was chatting to Diane.

"Morning, Diane!" I said cheerily.

"Good morning Michelle. How are you? Thanks so much for the party invite; did Nicky text you back?"

"I'm great, thanks," I answered. "Yeah, Nicky texted, that's no problem. Maybe next time?"

"Definitely!" said Diane. "Thanks again. Do you need to make your appointments for next week?"

We chatted a little more about the party as I booked in for my next few sessions, but it wasn't long before I was in real danger of being late. As I made my way towards the door, Ivan held it open in front of me.

"And they say chivalry is dead," I said with a smile as he walked me to my car. "You know, that was the second merciless torture session I've been subjected to in there this week. I think I should complain to the management. Oh wait, I am!" Ivan laughed at me. I winced as I raised my arm to place my bag in the back of the car. "Up to much today?" I asked him.

"Sort of," he said. "I'm here till around three, and then I have to collect my tux, get a haircut and meet the lads for dinner and drinks."

"Busy boy! Well, enjoy. I'd better get to work." I turned to get into my car.

"Give me a kiss!" Ivan blurted out.

I couldn't help laughing. "Oh my God! You are so romantic."

"Well, what was I meant to say?" he shot back with a cheeky grin. "You were leaving without giving me a kiss!"

I looked around the car park.

"What are you looking around for? We're consenting adults!"

"I know but there might be people from The Gym..."

"We *are* people from The Gym," he murmured, putting his arms around my waist. I leant towards him and we kissed. I melted away for what could have been a minute or could have been an hour, before becoming aware again.

"Okay," I said dreamily. "Okay. Yes. I've got to go now."

Ivan chuckled at my distracted demeanour.

"See you tomorrow, then. Enjoy your night."

I couldn't help it. I stood up on my toes and kissed him again before getting into my car, still a tad flustered. As I drove off, I felt grateful, excited and completely caught up in the flow. Life just seemed to be getting better and better. I arrived at work and spotted Fiona on her way in. I got out of the car and walked over to her.

"Hi, Fiona!" I said merrily. "How are you this morning?"

"Hi, Shelly! Not too bad, and you?"

252

"I'm great, thanks! Are you going to come to the party tonight?"

"Oh yeah," she said with conviction. "I replied to your email a few minutes ago. I'd love to come. I think Sarah is coming too, so we'll go together. I'm really looking forward to it. Who else will there?"

"Well, my sister Eve can't make it, she's in Galway. But there's Jake's sister Sam, Sam's friend Nicky, who also happens to be one of my trainers from The Gym, my Mum and Jake's Mum; I don't think Dee can make it but there are Sarah, Orla and yourself from work. Jen and Alice might be coming too, do you know them?"

"I know Jen. She's Martin's girlfriend, isn't she?"

"Yeah, that's her. She's a doll."

"I've heard of Alice, but I don't think I know her. That's Brian's girlfriend, right?"

"Spot on. She's lovely. She might be there tonight so you will get to meet her too. The girls from the band can't make it, unfortunately, as they have a wedding in Tipperary tomorrow night and they have to head there tonight to set up."

We continued chatting as we headed into the office, talking about the band, weddings in general, and my bespoke songwriting for tomorrow's big event. She loved the idea of having a brand new, original song for the first dance. After we got set up at our desks, she offered to go to the canteen for teas and coffees for everyone.

I realised I had forgotten to lodge the cheque, so I decided to take care of that at lunch. Everything else was in order, so I got straight to work and the morning went quickly. I didn't even look up from my desk until one o'clock when everyone else headed off for their breaks. I decided to pop up to see Mum, to check if she wanted to take a walk into town with me. As I approached the maternity ward, I saw her walking in the corridor. She invited me for a bite to eat and agreed to swing by the bank with me first.

We strolled in, and I express lodged the cheque into my account before we went to a little coffee shop for some lunch. It was good to catch up. I checked my phone before putting it on silent, then got stuck into the pile of work I'd left for myself, which I was determined to get finished before I left for the weekend. My phone buzzed as I got a text from Tracey.

*Just wanted to say thanks again for the song. We love it. I am singing it all the time. Pray, I don't get drunk on champagne and try to come onstage and sing it with you instead of dancing! I hear your dress is gorgeous on you. Hope you're coming to the whole wedding and enjoy the day. Wanted to say thanks again in case I don't get to see you before then. Tracey Xx*

I responded to Tracey's lovely message and then got properly stuck into work. I stayed completely focussed, and it was only when everyone started to get up from their desks to go home that evening that I became aware of the time. The girls came over to check if I needed them to bring anything with them later on.

"Just bring yourselves and your good mood or a drink to put you in a good mood," I advised.

After they'd all bustled out the door, I sat back in my chair and absorbed the uncharacteristic peace and quiet in the office for a few minutes before heading home and getting into party mode. I showered, ate and laid out my party clothes. As I was getting the food ready, the doorbell rang. It was Fionn.

We made our way into the living room and started setting up for a quick practice session.

"I've been playing around with the guitar style. I'd like to hear what you think," he said. "But I think we'll blow them all away. It's going to be awesome."

I laughed. I loved his confidence. He reminded me a little of Jake. We went over the song a few times, gave each other feedback and made a few adjustments. Then, we recorded it and listened back.

"Yup!" said Fionn. "I told ya we're amazing. That was easy."

I had a party to prepare for, and Fionn was meeting Aaron, Ivan and the rest of the lads for a few civilised drinks to commemorate Aaron's last night of being a bachelor. As he walked down the drive, Dad's car pulled up with Mum and Mary inside. I stood at the door to greet them. They hopped out of the car in full party mode, and I could tell Dad was relishing his chance to watch some sports at home in peace. I gave him a wave and he grinned from ear to ear as the ladies got to my door. He told us to have a good night, wished me luck for the wedding, and drove off with a look of contentment on his face.

Mum and Mary popped open a bottle of wine as soon as they got in the door, and started to help me to prepare the hot food. The doorbell rang, and it was Sam and Nicky. After a few minutes, the girls from work arrived, Alice and Jen. We all sat around the living room sipping our drinks and telling jokes and stories. I stood up from my chair and introduced everyone, just to break the ice a little more.

"Tonight is about fun!" I announced. "So, I'm going to feed you some finger food, leave ye get to know each other and have a few drinks. And then, the games will begin."

"What games?" Sam asked.

I looked at her with an air of mystery.

"Oh, you'll find out when it's time to find out," I grinned. "Okay so girls, drink away and have fun. I'll go get the food." I popped into the kitchen to get stuff ready and Jen followed me.

"Do you need a hand, Shelly?"

"Hiya Jen!" I said as I fiddled with a packet of pretzels. "That would be great, thanks. If you could just bring in some of these plates when I take the food out of the oven please."

"No problemo."

"So, Jen...how are you?"

"I'm fab thanks, Shell. You?"

"Oh, I'm great, thanks. Really great. Hey, I'm glad you and Alice came tonight. I haven't seen either of you in ages."

"I know. Well, since the funeral." Jen added.

"Well, yeah. I almost forgot that. We didn't really get to talk much, that day."

"Yeah, Alice and I were just saying that on the way over here. So..." she looked hesitant. "How are you really doing? I mean, don't get me wrong, I am really happy to see you happy. But, at the same time, I'm a little worried about you. You know...your sudden change of attitude and your other, I don't know how to put it, dramatic changes..."

I took a deep breath. I hadn't been expecting to have to talk about this.

"Okay, I can see why you'd feel that way. I know I haven't always been the easiest to get on with. You'd think, considering how close Jake and I were and how much I leant on him in general, that his passing would have killed me a bit too. I promise the reason I've started to change and I'm trying to enjoy life more is because...it's because Jake's death made me more aware of how precious life is. It took my best friend dying to make me see that I wasn't living..."

I trailed off. My voice had started to quiver. I could feel the tears start to glisten in my eyes and did my best to blink them away.

"Wow Shelly, you actually sound like Jake," Jen said softly. "I'm so sorry. I didn't want to upset you but I was beginning to think you were...you know?"

"In denial?" I finished for her, with my weepy voice. Tears started to flow down my cheeks as I took a deep breath. "Don't worry Jen. You and the rest of the girls...you're all thinking the same. I know you are. I'm not, though. I think about it every day" I said, squeezing out a smile. She gave me a big hug.

257

"Come on so, Shell. Let's just have a fun night. Just like you wanted, okay?"

I dried my eyes and composed myself.

"Yes. Let's." I took a deep breath and nodded, and we strode back into the living room with the food as if nothing had happened.

We brought the food into the room and we all sat around eating, drinking and playing party games. The food and drink were plentiful, and the company was exceptional. We ended up laughing all night long. I think in our own ways, we all needed it.

Eventually, Mary announced that she had to go and tottered a little unsteadily towards the door.

"Early start in the morning girls! Hair and makeup for the wedding! They won't do themselves!" My mum gave me a big hug and left with her, walking to the taxi office just around the corner. By half past midnight, the house was empty again and I was left to tidy up. Once the place was slightly less disorganised, I turned on the dishwasher and made my way to bed, thinking about how good all that laughter had been. I'd really enjoyed myself, apart from welling up in the kitchen with Jen. I'd started to bring more fun into my life, and I knew I wanted to keep it up. I fell asleep easily and after what felt like a split-second, I heard Jake's voice.

"That looked like a *hell* of a lot of fun," he said. "I was jealous I couldn't join in! They're a good old bunch, in fairness."

"Ya. It was a great night, Jake. I needed it. The new me needed it, even more, I think than the old me would have. I really feel the difference in my life since..." I paused for what seemed like forever, trying to frame what I was thinking until Jake said: "...since I died?"

"Well, yes. It sounds wrong, I know, but it's true."

"It seems like me dying is the best thing that ever happened to you."

"No, Jake! That's terrible! Don't *say* that."

"Relax, Shell," he said gently. "I may not be alive any longer but my sense of humour is. Are you okay?"

"Sorry," I said. "I know. I didn't mean to react like that. It's just that that tonight, I remembered that you...that after our time together like this is over, I won't see you anymore." I felt desperately sad, and Jake's face filled up with a look of profound sympathy.

"Shelly, I promise that the lessons you are learning, everything we're talking about, all these changes you're making, will guide you for the rest of your life. That'll be me being with you, every day. You won't see me, but I'll be right there. I've got your back. I've always had your back."

"I know, Jake," I said in a small voice. "I'm very grateful, you know. For everything. For all of it. Then and now."

"I know. But I want to help you to be you, not to be another me. You know that, don't you? Your life may take a very different path to mine because we *are* different. I remember hearing that a lot in the last few years: 'Not everybody's like you, Jake.'

"I used to think it was a bad thing but I learned to accept it for what it was."

259

"And what was it?"

"Not everybody's like me. Not everybody's like anybody! Not everybody's like you, or Mum, or Sam, or Michael, or my Dad, or your Dad, or your Mum, or your sisters, or your friends, or your workmates. Be yourself, Shelly. Everyone else is taken."

I laughed. Jake always had a way with words and he always knew how to cheer me up.

"So...let's take a look at a life we can both relate to, okay?"

"Let's!" I said brightly. I was anxious to elevate the mood. "Who?"

"Me. Born October 24$^{th}$, 1981, mother a wonderful woman, father a demon of a man. Two siblings; younger sister, older brother. Grew up with an alcoholic father, who created a war in our home on a regular basis. Lived on edge with Sam and Mike, wondering what would happen every time he walked in the door. Wondering when he'd start the next fight with Mam and what it would be about. Dinner not good enough? Shoes in the wrong place? Picture crooked on the wall? Anything could set him off and, if he had a drink in him, well, it just added fuel to the fire.

"Mike and I decided to stand up to him one day. I reckon Sam was probably only seven or eight years old. I was fourteen and Michael was sixteen. One day after school we stepped off the bus and we could hear screaming and shouting from inside the house. The back door was off the hinges, so we ran in. There in the kitchen was Pat, Mum and little Sam.

260

Sam was holding a knife to herself over at one side of the kitchen. Mum was sitting on the other side trying to coax her to drop the knife before she hurt herself. And there was Pat, standing over Mum, preventing her from getting up to help Sam, roaring and swearing at her.

I'll never forget that moment. Mike and I, without words, decided enough was enough. It was like we'd read each other's minds, so we charged at him, hit him as hard as we could and threw him to the floor. He'd been drinking – of course – so he wasn't that steady on his feet. As he fell...I always remember this detail and I don't know why...his glasses fell off and in that very moment, right then, I stopped being afraid of him. I actually felt sorry for him for a second. Then, Mum grabbed Sam and Michael and I just stood over him. We were getting big. I think we hadn't realised it until then.

"Mike looked down at him and said, 'you're getting old and you're getting feeble, and we're getting bigger and stronger and we've years left to go. We're not putting up with you anymore. Stop.' That was it. He just said 'stop' but not like a kid talking to his father. He said it...I don't know. Like a man. Like the guy in charge.

"Dad wasn't all that feeble, you know. A few minutes earlier, he was able to take the backdoor clean off its hinges. But Michael wasn't backing down, and neither was I. We stood together."

"And what happened next?" I asked, captivated and horrified. I'd never heard it before. I'd always known things got bad for the Lawlors, but I didn't know these details. Maybe nobody else did, apart from Mary, Mike and Sam.

261

Jake seemed uncharacteristically pensive. He stared off into the distance as he answered.

"The rest is history. Dad got sick shortly afterwards. He had cancer for nearly three years and then died. But after that day, he never started up so badly again. I think he just knew that if he did...I think he knew we wouldn't let him hurt our mother or our baby sister. I think he thought we might have killed him. I watched Mum care for him – out of obligation, more than out of anything else – and to be honest, I was glad when he was carted off to the hospice. He lived a very sad life, Shell, when he could have had a wonderful one."

Jake paused and sighed. Then he shook his head and looked up me again, more like his usual self.

"So? What am I trying to tell you?"

"Don't be a mean old drunk," I guessed.

"Well yeah, that too. But, if you look at my family, you see how we turned out and you begin to see that everything is a choice."

I could see what he was saying but I didn't think it was quite that simple.

"Not everyone thinks they have a choice, Jake."

He shrugged. "Maybe. But...did you ever meet my Dad's brother John? He lives in England with his family but they visit every few years."

"Oh yeah, I remember him. Really happy man. Head off your dad, but really nice."

"Yes, that's him. He's the perfect example. John and my father grew up with only two years between them. Same parents, same education, same opportunities, same capabilities and the same everything, pretty much. Dad turned out to be an abusive, mean, angry alcoholic while John turned out to be a kind, caring, funny, loving man. Why?"

"Luck," I responded hesitantly.

"No Shell. It's because not everybody is the same. And it's because what makes you who you are *is* up to you at some point. Not your parents, not your teachers, not your friends and not your circumstances. Michael or I could have become mean alcoholics, but we choose not to. We looked at our own experiences and made a choice."

"That's true..."

"You never know what's going on behind closed doors. Or in people's heads, for that matter."

Jake's heart-breaking story had made me think.

"It's strange, considering how much information is out there now. I mean you only have to look on Facebook and you can see what someone you went to school with ten years ago and haven't seen since is having for dinner, and where and with whom."

"Good point," Jake said. "As wonderful and useful as technology is, it has its drawbacks. I think people are losing their ability to communicate. They tell everyone the simplest, most uninteresting things you could imagine, but they won't tell you anything important. Nothing like 'I feel depressed' or 'I need help' or 'I'm lonely'. It's sad."

263

"That's true, too. It's a pity."

I looked at Jake, and for the first time in a while really appreciated what a wonder he was. Maybe because of his childhood and the path he chose, he developed better coping skills than most, but that was all down to his own force of will and his own desire to do as much good as he could in the world. He made a choice to learn from life and not to regret or hold onto things. That made him a happier person, and in turn, he made everyone around him a happier person. He could make someone a better person just by being their friend. That's what he'd done for me.

"It makes more sense to me now, you know," I told him. "Why you were so understanding and so forgiving. Why you were so good."

He smiled and shook his head just a little. Modest to the last.

"I started to hear 'not everybody's like you' differently and I realised it was a good thing. Nobody should try to be like anybody, that's what makes us all better. Jesus, Gandhi, Nelson Mandela...I could go on. They are all considered unique. They're all considered special. But they had people in their lives who said, 'not everybody's like you' too, and those people were right! And look at the differences they made. 'Be the change you wish to see in the world' - that's how Gandhi put it."

"Just remember that, Shelly. Not everybody's like you. In fact, nobody else is exactly like you. You're unique. The world was changed the second you arrived in it because nobody like you had ever been here before. Nobody like you will ever be here again. It's what you choose to do with your uniqueness that will really matter."

264

Unusually, we just sat together in silence for a while after that, just remembering what it was like to be in each other's company.

"Eighteen down," Jake said. "Three to go."

I woke up, and he was gone.

My eyes opened as if for the first time in my life. The winter sun shone through the skylight window and I could feel the little extra warmth it gave the room. I was happy. There was no worry, I didn't have any sense of being stressed or under pressure. I just felt good. "Is this how people are supposed to feel?" I wondered. I made my way downstairs, humming merrily to myself. It took me a little while to realise the melody was *Galileo*.

"I must remind Jake to tell me about that song and why it keeps popping up," I said out loud to myself as I ate breakfast and sipped my coffee. It was still early and I was in no rush, so I decided to go for an early morning walk before a nice, long, hot shower. I threw on some comfy clothes, then carefully laid the dress for the wedding on the bed and left for my appointment with the beautician.

I got my hair done in loose curls, my nails French-manicured and my makeup applied. By 12.30, I was ready for the wedding with plenty time to spare. I went home and got dressed before Michael picked me up. He was dropping Mary and me to the ceremony.

That dress fitted like a glove and I couldn't help admiring my shape in it. It wasn't all the dress, either; all of that time at the gym and my efforts to eat healthier food were really starting to pay off, too. I was pretty pleased with myself. Shortly after one o'clock, there was a beep outside. Punctual as always, there was Michael. I locked up the house and walked to the car. They both complimented me on how well I was looking. We all agreed that red, which I never usually wore, was definitely my colour.

We got chatting about the wedding, the bride and groom, and the song.

"I'm so glad you're getting back into songwriting," Mike said. "Well done! It's about time you got back into your original stuff."

I couldn't have agreed more.

"You're so right, Mike," I said. "I think I was probably a bit afraid of getting back into it, but now I feel like it's the right time in my life to write again. I don't want to procrastinate any longer. Better late than never!"

Michael looked over at me with an enigmatic smile.

"Do you know who you reminded me of just then?" he asked. I shook my head.

"Jake," he said. "It was like he was whispering in your ear."

That really made me smile, and I could see that Mary was smiling too. We chatted about this and that, and the lavish set-up Aaron and Tracey had organised for their big day, and Michael dropped us to the hotel just as a big crowd made their way inside through the side door.

The marriage was being held in one of the hotel's function rooms and Aaron and Tracey had a friend who was a celebrant, who'd be performing the ceremony. They had written their own vows and instead of

267

prayers, they had poems. A harpist played and a man with a beautiful tenor voice sang throughout the service. It was captivating.

I couldn't help but feel Ivan's eyes on me from time to time. I knew he was impressed by the dress. It was a big a change from my training gear or the oversized wetsuit, that's for sure. After the ceremony, the bride and groom left the room to have pictures taken in the garden, and Mary and I went straight to the bar to have a drink.

"Two glasses of champagne, please," Mary said without even waiting for me to hum and haw about whether I'd start drinking so early. She handed mine to me with a wink and a grin. I was feeling a little nervous, and I was really looking forward to getting my performance over and done with. Maybe a glass or two of bubbly would help to steady me.

"Wasn't that a lovely ceremony?" Mary said as she looked out over a sea of happy faces in every corner of the room. My mind was on the task that lay ahead, and when I didn't reply she gave my arm a squeeze.

"Shelly don't worry. It's only 4 o'clock and it's going to be quite late before you have to sing. Have a few drinks before dinner, enjoy yourself and relax. You'll be fine again."

She was right, of course. We sat at the bar sipping champagne and chatting until everyone was called into the main function room to wait for the bride and groom to arrive. We were seated with Tracey's Mum's friends and one or two of Tracey's friends. Mary introduced me to Tracey's Mum, Geraldine, while she was making the rounds to welcome the guests.

268

"Oh, you're the songwriter! Excellent!" she exclaimed when we were introduced. "I can't wait to hear this song. Tracey and Aaron have been raving about it all week."

"Oh God," I said, "That's a lot of pressure! I hope you'll like it now after all that!"

"Oh I will," she said with a laugh. "My Tracey knows what she likes. She has her mother's taste."

Just then, the bell was rung and we were all asked to be upstanding for the bride and the groom. They arrived to a torrent of applause, making their way through the crowd to the top table. Once we were all settled again, the first of six courses arrived and more wine was poured into our glasses by the omnipresent waiters. After the starters, we had a little break and the Best Man stood up to speak. One by one, the top-table crowd had their say.

By the time dessert was served, I was too full to even think about eating anymore.

"Mary," I said with concern in my voice, "I am going to burst out of this dress. I swear."

Mary was a little tipsy at that point, and she just laughed at me.

"Nonsense!" she giggled. "You don't have time to burst! You have to sing your song. You can burst out of it later when you're alone with handsome Ivan."

"Ha, ha, Mar, thanks for the advice," I responded sarcastically. "To be honest, I got slightly merry earlier but all that food sobered me right up."

269

"Me too, completely..." she said, except that the last word sounded more like "kupplitly". She gazed at me with a slightly goofy grin and blinked slowly.

"Ya right Mar! I think you could do with a cuppa, or I'll have to put you to bed before the band even starts."

She conceded the point, and we each stuck to tea for a few rounds. After the meal was over, they started to clear the tables and moved them aside to make the dance floor bigger. We relocated to the bar again, but as soon as we sat down I heard my name being called.

"Shell! Shell! Hey, how are you enjoying the day?" It was Fionn.

"Hey, Fionn!" I greeted him. "It's fab! We are having a ball. You?"

"It's great!" he said, looking around the room with a huge grin. He turned back to me and wiggled his eyebrows, saying in a conspiratorial tone "once we have the song done, I'll probably break out the shots."

"Are you not playing in the band?"

"Oh no. I have the night off. We have fillers for occasions like this."

"That's a good idea," I said approvingly. "You can just enjoy the night, so."

"Exactly. Anyway, I was wondering if you fancy doing a quick sound-check. Maybe up behind the stage?" It was a good idea. I made sure Mary was okay (she was nattering away to a group of friends with a tea in one hand and a champagne in the other; she was fine), and Fionn

270

and I headed towards the area behind the DJ box, next to the stage which had been set up for the band. Ivan, who I hadn't had a chance to talk to all day, seized the moment and ran over to say hi. Fionn grinned as he saw him approaching, and told me he'd be tuning his guitar and getting other things ready before he tactfully made himself scarce.

"You look absolutely gorgeous," Ivan said. "How's your day going?" I was aware that I was just staring at him, with wide eyes and what felt to be a fairly silly grin. I told myself to remain cool, calm and collected.

"My day has been great, really!" I answered. "Thank you for asking! How is yours?" I noticed that he was staring at me in exactly the same way, and that little detail alone was enough to make me want to sing.

"It's great, in fairness," said Ivan. "I think we're all ready to relax and just enjoy the rest of the night now."

"I think so," I agreed. "After the song is done, I can relax too." He laughed, and then looked almost sheepish as he realised that he was gazing at me. He tried to cover it up but failed miserably. I think he may have even blushed.

"Shell, I mean it, you know. You look amazing."

"Awh thanks, Ivan. You brush up pretty well yourself."

We spent the next few seconds just smiling at each other. It felt like an eternity. Eventually, it was Ivan who snapped us out of it, trying his best to return to cool, suave mode.

"Yes, well. I try. It's just part of the whole wedding thing, really, though. I'm actually very reserved and restrained, especially when it comes to things like this. Well, except if it's a sing-song at the end of a session. Then it's hard to shut me up usually."

"I'll be looking forward to that later," I said demurely. "But I'd better go and do my warm up with Fionn. I'll see you later."

Wordlessly, Ivan gently placed his hand on my lower back, pulled me towards him and kissed me. Then he winked, smiled his winning smile, and headed back into the throng as I walked behind the stage and joined Fionn for a quick check and run-through.

The music had started by the time I returned to Mary and her friends who had secured themselves a big table off to the side of the dance floor. It wouldn't be long before they called on the bride and groom to have their first dance. I decided to hold off on any more drinking until after the performance. I glanced around the room and noticed that everyone seemed relaxed and happy. Most people were chatting and laughing, with the exception of a few of the younger guests who were engrossed in their phones. More and more, people seemed to me to be living their lives through their phones. Even when in company, their phone seemed more important. Not more than a few feet away from me, two young women were sitting together at another table and both of them were playing with their phones. They weren't talking to each other or even looking at each other at all. At the table next to them were two older couples, who were chatting and laughing. The contrast was stark.

I was aware that I was looking around, taking a real interest in people, in what they were doing and in what their stories might be. I couldn't help but smile, as I thought of the massive differences in my life due to the changes in my outlook over those past weeks. I felt so grateful that I could have exploded. As I drifted off into my own world, the band paused in their setting up to make an announcement:

"Hey, everybody! Shortly, we will be welcoming the bride and groom to the dance floor for their first dance and they have an original first dance for you tonight. They have had their very own song written for their special day, and here to perform it live is the composer, Michelle Morrissey. Can we get a round of applause for Michelle please, with Aaron's brother Fionn Miller on guitar?" This was it. The moment of truth.

The guests all clapped as we made our way to the stage. I felt nervous, as usual, but there was a new feeling too, which seemed to be taking over. It was a feeling of confidence in myself. I sat at the piano and Fionn sat next to me on a stool. The lead singer of the band continued speaking, "Ladies and Gentleman. Will you please welcome to the dance floor for their first dance as husband and wife; Mr and Mrs Aaron and Tracey Miller?" We started playing the music as Tracey and Aaron walked into the room and onto the dance floor. Fionn and I started to sing.

> "*When the day comes and you find the one,*
> *there's a feeling that can't be denied.*
> *It's a feeling that you want to feel,*

*every day for the rest of your life.*

*And when the time's right,*

*You see it in their eyes*

*and you know you have all that you need.*

*And those magic moments, become magic days*

*and from days they turn to magic years.*

*So when you dance with me tonight,*

*I want everybody in the room to see,*

*that I'm the girl for you and you're the man for me,*

*and if our lives should end,*

*I want you to know that I could live a million lives,*

*and I'd still choose you as mine.*

*Some people spend their lives,*

*searching for what they believe is worthwhile.*

*But I know I've found that with you.*

*And no one can compare*

*because what we have is rare.*

*I know we make it that way, in all that we do.*

*So when you dance with me tonight,*

*I want everybody in the room to see,*

*that I'm the man for you and you're the girl for me,*

*and if our lives should end,*

*I want you to know that I could live a million lives*

*and I'd still choose you as mine.*

*So when you dance with me tonight,*

*I want everybody in the room to see,*

*that I'm the one for you and you're the one for me.*

*And if our lives should end,*

*I want you to know that I could live a million lives,*

*and I'd still choose you as mine.*

*So dance with me through life."*


As the music faded out, all the wedding guests were on or around the dance floor, they started to clap for the couple, and for Fionn and me. We left the stage and Fionn grabbed my hand. "Celebration time!" he declared. "Come on, Shell. We are doing a shot!"

We made our way to the bar as people shook our hands and congratulated us on our performance.

"What's it to be," asked Fionn, with his fingertips tapping on the smooth wood. I felt a little apprehensive.

"Oh...I don't know about shots, Fionn."

"What do you mean, you don't know? You just performed a song you wrote and everybody loved it! Now you get to celebrate and enjoy the night. Come on; one shot. Live a little. Have some fun."

The word 'fun' hit me like some kind of trigger. My mind was made up. It was shot o'clock.

"Okay. Sambuca."

"Perfect," said Fionn with approval. "My favourite. Two Sambucas please."

We drank the shots straight back and broke out laughing and spluttering. Fionn turned to me.

"Oh, by the way, Michelle, I have to say you're looking amazing. Ivan is a lucky guy."

"Aw, thanks, Fionn," I said with a smile. "You look very dapper yourself."

Fionn gave me a mock salute, slammed his shot glass down on the bar, and headed back over to where his friends were gathered. I made my way back to Mary's table. She gave me a huge hug told me how proud she was of me. Jake, she said, would be smiling down on me like a proud big brother. I desperately wanted to tell her that I knew he was proud and to tell her how I knew, but I couldn't. Instead, I just squeezed her hand and smiled at her. She looked up as someone stood behind me, and then a familiar voice asked me to dance.

"I suppose I can squeeze one dance with you before the queue gets any bigger, Ivan. I have a waiting list, you know." Mary tried to wink subtly, patting me dramatically on the leg before turning back around to the girls for what looked to be some particularly enjoyable gossip.

Ivan and I walked to the dance floor. Aaron and Tracey were still giving it their all, and they smiled at us as we arrived. Tracey shouted "oh yeah, typical Ivan! Picks the most popular girl in the room!"

"Second most popular, babe," Aaron added. "Michelle, again, from the bottom of our hearts, thank you so, so much for all the work you put in. It was one of the high points of the day so far. And, just because

276

we like you, you can have our Ivan. No charge. Be sure to read the instruction manual."

We all laughed and threw ourselves into dancing for a few songs. After a while, Ivan leant over to me. "Do you fancy a drink, Shell?" he asked sweetly.

I hadn't had one of those in about ten minutes, so it was high time for a refill. We left the dance floor, sat at the bar with our drinks, and just talked.

"What are you doing tomorrow night, Shell?"

"I don't have any plans, really. Probably nurse a hangover!"

Ivan asked the barman for a glass of water and placed it in front of me.

"In between each drink, have a glass of water and you will be perfect tomorrow. There's no better way to stave off a hangover."

"You're right, and I will." I drank half the glass of water in one go. "So what's happening tomorrow night?"

"A surprise," Ivan replied.

"Really? A surprise date? What a good idea! Only a genius would come up with an idea like that!"

"I know," he answered. "I *am* a genius. What can I say? So, be ready at 7 pm and I'll pick you up."

"Should I dress up or stay casual?"

"Dress up. It's not an activity. That's all I am going to say about it."

"Fair enough, Ivan. That means it's your job to ensure that I don't get too drunk and end up hung-over. Okay?"

"Okay, will do."

We danced and chatted for hours and, at the end of the night, the last of the wedding party started to move into the resident's' bar. I began to feel unwell and I made a discreet exit to the ladies toilet. No sooner had I entered the cubicle, then everything I had eaten and drank all day made a surprise reappearance. Luckily, I was alone in the toilet and after vomiting for a good five minutes, I attempted to get up but I failed. I fell back onto the toilet seat. I was far, far drunker than I'd thought.

"Michelle Morrissey," I slurred to myself, "I really thought you'd moved passed this part of your life. I thought you were beyond drinking till you got sick and passed out in the bathroom. You're an adult!"

I closed my eyes for a second to try to clear my head, and when I opened them again, I was startled to find that I was crammed into the cubicle with Jake. My heart sank.

"Ah Jesus, Jake! Don't tell me I fell asleep in the bloody toilet!"

"Well...it's not all that bad," he said in a calming voice I remembered from a hundred other drunken nights where he'd been my voice of reason. "In fact, it could be a lot worse."

"Worse? Worse! Worse in...How? How could it be worse, Jake? I'm asleep in the toilet! Ivan is out there with no idea where I've gone. It gets worse? It doesn't get worse! Please explain!"

I was very distraught.

278

"I should never have drunk that Sambuca. Those Sambucas. How many Sambucas did I have? I had too many Sambucas, Jake. Jake, what will I do? Ivan is here! I've ruined everything! I...oh my god...am I on the floor?! Please tell me I'm not on the floor!"

"Relax, Shell," said Jake, confidently. "It'll be fine. You didn't get sick on yourself, or on your dress. You are in fact asleep sitting bolt upright on the toilet seat and when you wake up, remember that you're going to feel fine. You were smart enough to bring your handbag, so you can touch up your makeup, and you have some chewing gum and a bottle of nice perfume. You'll be good as new."

I looked up at Jake from the toilet seat. He was leaning against the door with a beaming smile. He clearly thought that this was hilarious.

"I feel better now," I grumbled. "Thanks."

"No problem, Shell. That's what I came back for: to make your life easier and better. Remember?"

"Yeah. Heart of gold. So nobody's going to know I was in here getting sick?"

"No, but in any event, haven't I told you a million times? What others think of you is none of your business!"

I grumbled at him again. I may have hiccupped.

"Shell, you're the only person who needs to think about you. In the real world, people don't actually think about other people all the time because they're too busy thinking about themselves. We're harder on ourselves than anybody could ever be when really, we should be nicer to ourselves than anybody could ever be. If we all started to take responsibility for ourselves and work on improving our opinions of who we are, we'd be a lot better off. Instead, we give all that control to others."

I looked up at him through one bleary eye, squinting the other against the harsh light in the cubicle.

"What on earth are you on about?" I sighed.

"Whenever you blame someone for something that happened to you, you give them all the power. You weren't happy at work and you kept blaming your boss, your work colleagues, and your job and all the rest of it. You did nothing about it for ages. You can't change your boss or your colleagues, but you can change you. What's happened at work since you decided to change?"

He was right. Things were much better at work, and nothing had changed except my attitude. Jake kept driving his point home.

"Relationships, then. In relationships, it usually starts out all happy and lovely and all that like you and Ivan are now. Then, over time, it can begin to get a little...umm..."

"Boring?" I suggested.

"People who are bored are boring people, Shell. But, yes that's exactly it. We look for something or someone to blame. We start to look at all the things that our partner does that annoy us, and we totally forget all the wonderful things that attracted us to them or caused us to fall in love with them. The only solution is ourselves and how we look at them."

"So, we're the problem, Jake? Everybody? People?"

"Yes, we are."

"Okay. But if we're the problem, we're also the solution, right?"

280

"Right, Shell. That's what I mean by 'don't give the power away'. That's like giving your friend the remote to the TV and expecting them to know what you want to watch, then getting annoyed if they don't put that on. The simple solution would be to just put on what you wanted."

It made a lot of sense.

"I used to get really mad at guys when they didn't do the things to make me happy," I agreed. I tried to think of an example.

"Like...reading my mind. Is that too much to ask?"

Jake laughed, "Yeah, tell me about it!" I thought about all the times I'd been snappy with Jake for no reason. A wave of guilt threatened to wash over me, but I held it together.

"I know you put up with that, Jake, but I didn't realise what I was doing. I can see now, though. I feel a greater...I don't know what you'd call it. An understanding, I suppose, now more than ever, about myself."

Jake looked at me with such an expression of love and affection that I almost wept.

"You really, really have. I'm so proud of you. I'm so happy you've been willing to learn so much in 16 days. You're a new woman! I had my doubts, you know? But now, I know that you have all the tools you need to go forward, and to keep going forward."

"I feel good, Jake. And I can't believe it's been over two weeks. The time has passed so quickly."

"Yes. You only have two sleeps left, Shell."

281

"I know," I said. It made me sad to think about. "But we'll make the most of it, yeah?"

"We sure will, Shell. Just try not to pass out in the toilet again in the next 24 hours!"

We laughed.

"Do you remember the first night after I came back, Shell?

"I do. You told me about the hall with the thousand mirrors."

"Do you think that you understand that a little better now?"

"I do. I'm the first dog, these days."

"What you see in others, you have in yourself. You can only give away what you have. Be happy, and you'll see happiness everywhere and you can show everyone else. Be angry, and you'll see anger everywhere. When you give that out, that's all you get back. Now..." he said, "...as much as I'd love to stay and chat some more, there's someone out there who wants to spend time with you just as much as I do. It's time to wake up. Enjoy the rest of your night."

I awoke with a bit of a start, somewhat uncomfortable perched atop the toilet seat. I fixed myself up, walked out of the cubicle to the sink, washed my hands and took a chewing gum from my bag. Then I applied lipstick and eyeliner and finished with a spray of perfume. As I walked back into the resident's' bar, I met Mary in the corridor. She'd been looking for me. Michael was on his way to pick her up and she offered me a lift.

"Thanks, Mary. I'll just pop over to Ivan and let him know. I'll be back to you in five minutes."

I tracked Ivan down quickly and told him I was about to head away. He looked crestfallen.

"You can't leave now!" he protested. "There's a sing-song about to start. Besides you can stay in my room."

I laughed out loud at the idea. He gave me a haughty look.

"I have two beds in my room so don't get carried away," he laughed. "Besides, I'm not that easy. I respect myself more than that."

As weak as his argument was, I think it's what I'd been hoping to hear. "Okay then," I said. "I'll stay." I went back to Mary and told her to go ahead without me, and she wiggled her eyebrows lasciviously, swearing that wouldn't say anything to my mother or my father. I rolled

283

my eyes at her with a smile and gave her a hug before she went on her way. Then, I returned to the bar and sat down next to Ivan.

It wasn't long before the sing-song began. Fionn had his guitar out and sang a few requests. There were two other guys with guitars and they sang and played too. After a while, Tracy got to her feet and Aaron shouted for the noble call, holding his arms out for silence. He regretted it a moment later, though when she asked him to sing *Isn't She Lovely?* Still, he pushed through it with gusto, serenading his new wife. He sung 'Isn't she lovely?'

Once Aaron had finished doing his best Stevie Wonder impression, he called on Fionn.

"Sing *Galileo*," he said to his little brother. Fionn obliged, and as he did I noticed Ivan singing along in a low voice. He stopped when he saw me looking, and turned to me.

"Do you like Declan O'Rourke?" he asked.

"I love him," I said truthfully. "He's a great musician. I take it you do too?"

"Yup. He's a legend."

After Fionn finished and the clapping was over, it was Fionn's turn to call. He fixed his eyes on me and pointed. "Shelly!" he shouted. "Shelly for a song!"

I'd partly guessed this was coming so I asked for a guitar and played *Last Request*. Several songs and drinks later, Ivan leant over and murmured in my ear "it's well past my bedtime, Shell. Are you tired?"

It was four in the morning. It was definitely time to hit the hay. I followed Ivan to the lift and fell into his arms as he hit the button for his floor. When we got to the room, I threw myself onto the only bed there.

"Oh ya, two beds is it Ivan? I'm onto you!"

Ivan lay down next to me and we kissed each other in the dark. We were both tired, though, and before long, I realised I was lying in bed with both Ivan and Jake.

"Well, this is awkward," said Jake. "I've never been part of a threesome before."

I sat up like I got an electric shock. "Oh My God! Jake! What's going on?"

"Relax Shell. You're asleep. I'm dead. I thought you would have the hang of this by how. "

Jake turned his eyes to Ivan.

"He's fast asleep too, so no need to panic. All is well."

My memory of the last hour or two of the night was a little fuzzy. Jake noticed me looking at Ivan and trying to piece together the last few minutes before I'd fallen asleep.

"Shell, you're both lying on top of the bed covers and all of your clothes are on. Relax."

I breathed a sigh of relief. I didn't want things to move too fast with Ivan. I had a feeling there was more going on between us than quick thrills, and I hoped he'd be willing to invest the same time I was.

"Did you enjoy your day?" Jake asked.

"I had a wonderful day," I said. "The wedding was so nice and so original. They wrote their own vows and had poems instead of prayers. The music was fabulous, so was the food. It was the best wedding I have ever been to."

"That's great!" said Jake. "Do you maybe think that you were the difference that made your experience better today?"

"Well, I did have a really nice thought earlier about how happy I am. And I did feel a new kind of confidence that's almost…" I cast around for the right word. "It's almost familiar if that makes sense."

"Yes, it does. Perfect sense."

"I have so much I want to do now, Jake. I'm so much more aware of what I need to change. I've wasted so much time and I really want to make the most of everything now. I want to do more things, see more places and have new experiences. I want to do all the things I only dreamed of up to recently."

Jake nodded in approval, with a look of pride on his face. Then, he turned to me and said: "How do you build a wall?"

"Uh…what?" I replied, a little bit blindsided by the random question.

"How do you build a wall?" he repeated.

"Ah, no, I don't know Jake. I haven't a clue how to build a wall."

"It's easy!" he declared. "One brick at a time!" All of a sudden his weird question made sense. I apologised for not getting the point.

"It's okay," Jake chuckled. "It's the little distances that get you to your destination, even on the longest journey. A to B to C to D…all the way to Z. You build brick by brick. It's good to know where you want to go, but you also need to know how to get there. Where you are going on your next holiday."

"Em... I don't know, probably Canada."

"Perfect. That's the hard part done; the decision. What do you do next to make that happen?"

"I book a flight."

"Then what?"

"I tell my sister I am coming and book time off work."

"And?"

"I suppose I'd pack and maybe order currency."

"How do you get your flight?"

"I go to the airport."

"Yes, Shell. How do you get there?"

"I probably get a lift off Dad or a taxi."

"Can you see how many little things that you never even consider are all part of a bigger goal? Rome wasn't built in a day, but a bit of it was." Jake paused, taking the time to look around the room. He sat up and folded his arms, looking as if he were inspecting the scene. "So, this is cosy," he said. "You, me and Ivan the Great. Three in the bed and the little one said?" He made a point of being very amused by the whole scenario.

"Jake, on a serious note."

"A serious note? Do you think this is the time or the place?"

"Yes, I do. This is sleep twenty, isn't it?"

"Yes, Shell. It is."

"So...after tomorrow night, are you really going to be gone? Or, will you ever come back? You know, randomly? Like, if I need you or...or...if you're bored, or if you need me, or something? Or anything?" I didn't want my friend to go. I didn't want to miss him again. I remembered my heartbreak at his funeral. I was terrified that I'd have to go through it all again.

"Michelle..." Jake looked serious, and even a little sad. He reached down and held my hand. "After tomorrow night, I will not only be gone from your life but I will be gone from your sleep...except maybe for dreams. I will not be appearing in this way again. If you do have a random dream of me, it will be a projection of your thoughts and experiences. I'm moving on. I have to. I have to go, and there's no coming back. If there's anything that you want to ask me, if there's anything you want to say or to hear me say, your next sleep is your last chance. It's *our* last chance."

I could feel tears welling up again, but I pushed them away with sheer force of will. I didn't want Ivan to wake up and find me crying in my sleep while I lay there next to him.

"Jake?" I asked in a small voice. He squeezed my hand as I looked up at him. "I need to know...why have I heard *Galileo* so much since you've died? What does it mean? It's in my head, or it's on the radio, or it's on the television, or Ivan is singing it or..." Jake interrupted me mid flow.

"I promise, I'll tell you tomorrow, okay?

"Okay," I whispered.

"You went to bed very late. This is going to be a short sleep. You and Ivan are about to wake up. Remember, won't you? Remember the little bricks, and all the little changes make the big differences."

My eyes opened, and it was just me and Ivan. He'd turned over in the bed and woken me up. He reached up and touched my face as he did his best to focus.

"How's the head?" he asked.

"My head's fine," I said. "How about yours?"

"Tender. Very tender. But all in all, I think I'll survive." He rubbed his eyes and looked at his watch "Nine o'clock. Sunday morning, 10$^{th}$of November 2013."

"Thanks for the in-depth update, Big Ben," I said sarcastically.

He chuckled, then stretched out with a huge yawn. I snuggled into him as he did.

"Breakfast?" he asked. As soon as he mentioned it, I realised I was famished. After all, I'd managed to throw up just about everything I'd eaten the day before and there'd been nothing to fill the gap afterwards except for a few more drinks.

"Yes!" I said emphatically. "But I'm not eating anywhere dressed like this." Ivan sat up on the bed and looked at me.

"What do you mean? You look beautiful!"

"I'm sure I do, but this is last night's party dress, not today's breakfast outfit! I will not be seen eating breakfast in shame." He conceded the point.

"Okay, so how about I pop in the shower and change, then I'll drop you home to change, and then I'll take you for the best breakfast in town?"

"That sounds like a plan, Batman."

"Okay, Robin. Give me ten minutes, okay?"

After a quick shower, Ivan checked out and we drove to my house. He waited downstairs while I showered and put on some normal Sunday clothes.

We went for breakfast at the Coffee Dock and chatted and laughed about the wedding and all the things that had happened the night before. After a few hours, he dropped me home and we kissed goodbye, reminding me about our date that night.

"I'll pick you up at 7 pm, okay?"

"Perfect. See you then. Have a good day."

As he drove off, I waved goodbye. Sunday was off to a great start. I couldn't wait to see how it would turn out.

Chapter 21 - Sleep 21

*Sunday 10<sup>th</sup> November*

Around noon, I decided to visit my family. I really wanted to see Eve so I could fill her in on the weekend. It was another beautiful day, so I decided to walk and enjoy the fresh air. I grabbed my jacket, gloves and scarf and started the 20-minute stroll. While walking, I thought of how short my time had been with Jake on the last visit and how that night would be the last time I would see him again. I wondered what I should ask him. I felt confident that I understood what he had taught me over the past twenty visits. I also knew that it was fine to intellectually understand the things he had said and to be inspired by them but it was a whole another thing to take action. Jake had said that to me repeatedly, and I could think of plenty of other examples in my own life too.

When I arrived at my parents' house, there was no car in the driveway. I went around the back and opened the door. I walked in and there was no one to be seen. I made my way to Eve's bedroom and I crept in quietly. Eve was sound asleep.

The only remedy, I decided, was to take a flying leap and land right on top of her. I pounced, like a slightly hungover jungle cat. Eve shouted some pretty colourful words and called me some pretty impressive names, but in the end, she was defenceless in the face of my

291

ninja attack. Eventually, she stopped swearing and instead used the magic word.

"PLEASE stop jumping on me!" she whimpered. I relented.

"You're a spoilsport. I was having so much fun." Slowly, Eve poked her head out from under her quilt. Her eyes were squinty little slits and she looked as if she'd been just thrown into bed by an angry giant.

"What's wrong?" I asked. "Are you not having fun? Are you hungover?"

"Yes!" she shouted. "God damn it, yes! I thought you were at that wedding yesterday. Why aren't you hungover too? That's what normal people are like the day after a wedding!"

"Little sister," I said in my best sensei voice, "you have much to learn. You must follow my teachings."

Eve seemed less than enthusiastic about my teachings. I sat next to her in the bed.

"Where are Mum and Dad?"

"They are gone to the graveyard and then I think they're going for lunch somewhere."

"That explains that, then," I said. "So, how was your weekend away? When did you get back?"

"Late last night, then I went straight out. I only got home around eight this morning. What time is it now?"

"It's just after one o'clock."

"Ugh," she said disapprovingly as she glared at me. "Thanks for the wake-up call, you waggon. I was hoping to make it all the way through to tomorrow morning. Ok then, seeing as you simply had to wake me, you're clearly bursting to give me some sort of gossip or scandal. Go on. Spill it."

I filled Eve in on all that had been happening, from surprise date number one with Ivan to my fun party at home with the girls, to the wedding, and the singing, and the drinking, and spending the night in Ivan's room. That brought us right up to current events and surprise date number two that night.

"You seem to have done more in the past few days than you've done in years," she said, and she seemed genuinely impressed. "No offence," she added.

"Oh, none was taken. You're right. I have, and it's been fun. I feel like a teenager again."

"What are you going to wear tonight?"

I hadn't even considered that yet.

"That's a good point," I told her. "I have absolutely no idea. What do you think I ought to wear?"

"Good question," she sighed. "Clearly, you need my help. We're only as good as the questions we ask"

"Who said that?" I asked. I liked that little aphorism.

"What do you mean who said it? I said it. You just heard me."

"Yeah," I said, "but whose quote is it originally?"

"Me, you dope," she said, indignant. "That's an Eve Morrissey original. They're very valuable. Now, let's dress you to impress."

We spent another hour looking through Eve's wardrobe. She drank several cups of coffee, and I tried on loads of clothes. Eventually, we agreed on an outfit. I stood in front of the full-length mirror in her room, admiring myself. I was wearing stonewashed skinny jeans, brown knee-high boots, a cream blouse, a brown belt and a tweed blazer.

"I really like this outfit," I said to Eve. "I never seen you wear any of these."

"I've never worn them together. I like it too, actually. I probably will wear it as an outfit after you now." We made a few more small adjustments to some accessories while Eve had yet another coffee, and before too long it was time for me to make a move. I promised Eve I'd text her with details about the mysterious destination as soon as I knew them, then headed out the door.

On the walk home, I called Mary to see how she was handling her morning-after head. She sounded pretty ill, but very happy. She'd had a great time. When I arrived home, I got my clothes ready for the gym and work the next day, then I showered and started to get ready for my hot date.

At seven on the button, I heard a beep outside. I put on my jacket, grabbed my handbag and checked myself in the mirror one last time before hurrying out the door. I couldn't believe how much I was looking forward to seeing Ivan after just a few hours.

He was much improved from this morning, bright-eyed and full of life. I tried to get him to tell me where we were going but he held firm, insisting that it was going to be a surprise. However, he'd never come up against my insistent nature before. After a solid five minutes of pestering, he broke enough to tell me that we were going to go and see a show. Once he realised that I was about to move on to phase two of the pestering to find out where he pre-empted me by telling me that it was at the Opera House.

I had no idea who was playing. Ivan grinned at me good-naturedly, and he seemed glad that I'd decided to not pester him any further. As a reward, he started giving me tiny clues on the drive in. Eventually, after a few confused minutes, I had a flash of insight and the penny dropped.

"Oh my God!" I gasped. "It's not Declan O'Rourke, is it?!" Ivan's grin was as wide as the Cheshire cat's.

"Maybe!"

"Really? I mean, really really?"

"Would you be pleased if it was?" he asked.

I was filled with excitement and could barely stop myself from jumping up and down in my seat.

"Yes, I would. That would be amazing, Ivan! Completely amazing!"

Ivan smiled, "I made a good call then."

I dove over the gear lever and the handbrake and gave him a big kiss on the cheek.

"Thank you so, so much," I said. "This is wonderful. It really is. In fact, I can't think of a better way to end the week."

"Easy!" he laughed. "I'm trying to drive here!" I just about managed to restrain myself for the rest of the short drive into the city. "Just remember who you came here with tonight," Ivan told me as he parked. "Don't be running off with Declan."

We got to the bar and Ivan ordered a water himself and a glass of wine for me. Our seats were in row F, very close to the stage. The show began with a support act, a young girl with a guitarist who performed a few original songs. Then, Declan and his mini-orchestra came to the stage and, from 9 pm to 10.30pm, they didn't leave. He played right through with no breaks, jumping from guitar to piano, and playing old favourites as well as brand-new songs I'd never heard before.

As I sat there taking it all in, I thought of Jake and how much he lived for these kinds of special moments. As kids, all we wanted was to be in a band and be famous. As teenagers, we wanted to do nothing more than go to gigs all the time. The more I thought of him, the more real it all became. That deep, anxious sadness rose up again, in spite of my surroundings. After that night, I'd never see Jake again.

*Galileo* was, of course, inevitable. It came at the very end of the night. As Declan sang Jake's favourite song, I listened as if I'd never heard it before. Jake was in every word of it. There was a comfort and beauty to that thought which hadn't occurred to me until then, but as I listened to the song unfold, I knew that whenever I felt lonely and missed Jake, I could always listen to it and feel like he was with me. As the orchestra held the final note, I realised I had tears in my eyes.

"Are you okay, Shell?" Ivan asked. I could hear the concern in his voice.

"Oh, ya. Sorry, Ivan. It's just...*Galileo* was Jake's favourite song. It just reminds me of him." He hugged me tightly for a few minutes until nearly everybody else had left the auditorium. As we got up to follow them through the ornate doors at the back, I couldn't resist the urge to pull his arm around my shoulder.

"Thank you so much," I said, looking up into his big, beautiful eyes.

"You're welcome," he smiled back down at me. "Next surprise date is your turn."

"My, aren't you the presumptuous one?" I said with mock indignation.

"I am," he agreed. "But that's only because I know what I want." I held my head up, confidently.

"I have plenty of surprise dates up my sleeve, Ivan. Don't you worry!"

He dropped me home, we kissed goodnight, and Ivan waited until I was in the door before driving away. After a wonderful, if somewhat full-on weekend, I was exhausted. I made my way upstairs and into bed. As I lay there, I started to think about all the questions I wanted to ask Jake but one kept repeating in my mind as I drifted off to sleep.

"It's our last visit together and I must say the past few weeks...you've amazed me, Shelly. I always had faith in you, but I've seen you flourish more since the funeral than in all the years I knew you. I'm really, really proud of you."

"It's all because of you," I said, facing into my pillow. I didn't want to turn around and look at him. I wasn't sure I'd be strong enough to do it without crying and begging him not to go. "I feel like life has so much to offer, now. I feel alive again. Oh...I'm sorry Jake," I said, afraid of upsetting him.

He just laughed, "That was a quick recovery." I felt him sit at the edge of the bed. "I was going to ask you what it is you had been thinking about asking me. However, we both know that I already know that so...just ask." I took a deep breath and forced myself to sit up and look him in the eye.

"Why?" I said. "Why?! Out of all the people you could have come back to help, like your Mum, or Sam or Michael...why did you come back to me? What made me more in need of you than any of them?"

Jake sighed and looked down at his hands. The silence, while he thought about exactly what to say, seemed to go on for hours. When he finally looked up at me again, it was with the most bittersweet, gentle smile I'd ever seen on his face in all the years we'd known each other.

"Because if I didn't, you would have been my one 'I shoulda'."

I didn't know what that meant. I didn't know what to say. I just looked at him.

"Remember at my funeral, you quoted me in your eulogy?" Jake asked. "You said 'Jake always said he didn't want a load of 'I shoulda's' at the end of his days.' You were right. I...I didn't want to be able to say I should have helped you, to know that I *could* have helped you, but I didn't. I didn't want to spend my time doing whatever is next thinking 'I wish I could have helped my best friend Shelly to find her own way to happiness." Jake paused waiting for me to respond.

"Thank you, Jake" I barely managed to say. "Thank you for not giving up on me. Thank you for never giving up on me. Thank you for coming back and giving me a chance to say thank you. Thank you for everything."

"What are best friends for?" he asked me simply. "Best friends carry each other through the tough times and walk side by side through the good times."

I reached out for Jake and hugged him as tight as I could. We stayed like that for a long time.

"How can you just accept this?" I asked eventually. "Why just 21 days? How can you just calmly say you have to go when you managed to find your way back? Why aren't you mad that you're dead?! You were just 33 years old. That's all! You were just 33! Are you not angry that you had so much more to give, so much more to *be*, and that it was all just taken away? That you were taken away from all of us?"

"No Shell. I'm not. Where I am now, there's no anger, there's no sadness, and there's no suffering. We pass on, but we don't die the way people imagine it. I'm not sure how to explain it to you. I wish I did, but I really don't. It's not that you wouldn't understand, it's that you literally can't until you get here. It's...it's about energy. You can't create it. You can't destroy it. You can just change it. That's what happened to me.

I was changed. The closest I can come to is...I think maybe 'transcended' is the closest thing to it. We transcend into bliss. It actually is bliss and I understand the meaning of the word now. There is no worry, no pain, and no struggle. It's just...joy. Pure joy and complete love."

"Okay," I said. "Okay. I think I can understand. I just wish you could have had more of your life here. You were a good man, Jake. You were maybe the best man I knew. It's not fair that you only had a little while to share yourself with people."

"Shelly," Jake said earnestly, "life's for living. It's just an experience; one of many. Once you understand that, you're free to see it for what it really is. You get me?"

"I do."

"I'm not the only person who's come back like this. It happens more than you might think. Sometimes, we're dismissed as dreams or delusions. Sometimes the people we want to talk to can't accept what's happening and never see or hear us at all. If you're open to a sign you will get one. But you know the real reason you don't hear more about it, don't you."

"I think so."

"Tell me."

"Because I can't tell anyone about it. It's a secret. That's part of the deal, isn't it? It's our secret."

"Yes, that's part of the deal. Besides, if you did tell people, they'd only worry about you! Go through your life with your eyes open and see everything, Shelly. That's what matters. Do you remember when 'The Squire' died?"

"Yes Jake, I remember. Amazing man."

"Yes, he was. Do you remember, for about a year after his death, I was having dreams about him? In my dream, he was alive and I was afraid to call to his house and I kept passing by? I was terrified; do you remember?"

"Yes, I do. You said it seemed like he was calling you."

The Squire had been Jake's grand-uncle; Mary's Uncle John. He had been a local legend. My Dad had told me that when he was young, one of the first things anyone would say if something had gone seriously wrong was 'get The Squire.' He was the type of man who always knew what to do; a gentle, ancient soul. When he died, the whole community practically shut down.

"His death was hard on all of us," I continued. "He was like Santa Claus to the rest of us, but I know you and he were very close. He was like a father to you."

"He was Shell, and he was one of my greatest teachers. But back to the dreams. I had been having them for ages and one night when I was in Martin's place, his mum Dol, you know Dolores, right?"

"Of course! I love her!"

When we were small, we called Dolores "Angel Lady." She did tarot readings, fortune telling, horoscopes and all the rest but more importantly, she was just a lovely, kind, caring lady who always had time for everybody, in spite of the cruel life she lived at the hands of her husband.

"Not long after The Squire went, after he died, I mean, I was over at Martin's. Dol was sitting on the floor by the fire. She told me to sit down by her. She passed me the cards. She told me to shuffle them and to think a question I wanted to have answered. So, she did her thing and then said the cards were saying 'talk' or 'answer'. She asked me if it made sense. I told her it didn't.

"But, then Martin interrupted and said, 'what do you mean 'no'? You keep dreaming that The Squire is alive and that he's trying to talk to you, so it sounds like you need to talk back!' Dol asked me about the dreams. I explained to her that I had been dreaming about him being alive and waiting for me in his big old chair, where he used to always sit, but I wouldn't call into the house. Something was holding me back. I always dreamed that he was speaking to me, but that I couldn't quite understand what he was saying. I think that's what I found scary...not being able to make out the words,

"Then, Dolores said something that made sense at the time and makes, even more, sense now. She said that maybe me not calling in to see The Squire was me refusing to listen to him and that maybe he was hanging around to get my attention. Maybe he was trying to give me a sign."

"And?" I asked Jake.

"So...I listened. I went home that night and I was reading a book...I can't remember what, but the bookmark was a little memorial thing for The Squire. It had that story 'Footprints' on it...you know the one where a man walks along a beach with God and looks back over his life, and sees that at the worst times, there's only one set of prints?"

I knew the story.

"Yes," I told Jake. "The man says 'look at all those bad times, when I was so hurt and so lonely when there's only one set of prints! Why did you abandon me when I needed you most?!' and God says 'I love you and I never left you...those are all the times I carried you'."

"Yes, that's the one. So...that night, when I dreamed about The Squire calling me from his house, I didn't run past like I always had. I went in. I sat down. I talked to him. And...do you know what happened?"

"He talked back," I answered.

"For 21 nights," Jake said. "That is why I know, that when you really believe, you will receive. I was very open-minded, but I still didn't understand what was going on until Dol and Martin helped me. Imagine how often we try to come back and nobody can help, and our messages are never heard! That's how I knew I could come back to you. I just...I don't know how to describe it. I *asked.* And suddenly there I was, talking to you. I think I was allowed back because I knew I really had a chance to try to help you to be happy and it was my deepest wish."

I was taken aback that Jake loved me so much, in spite of all my faults that his greatest wish, his *last* wish, was to help me to simply learn how to be happy. I knew I could never thank him enough, but I could show him my gratitude by living up to the faith he'd had in me.

303

"Jake...you did it. I am so much happier now and I know, without any doubt, that I can create and control my own happiness. I know that it's better to go for the things that scare me rather than wonder 'what if?' It will all work out in the end and if it doesn't work out, it's not the end."

"I like that Shell," he said. "Very nice. And, I think I'm in a good position to say, very true. Shell, some people spend their whole life searching for the meaning of life, but there's only one meaning. The funny thing is, everybody, realises it at some point but it amazes me how many still keep searching, still keep asking, questioning, analysing and overcomplicating the answer."

"So?" I asked. "What's the meaning of life?" His cheeky grin returned.

"Isn't it obvious? The meaning of life is to live and be happy! See all you can see! Do all you can do! That's why we are here. And, we're here to learn from every experience. They're all bricks in the wall. They're all steps on the way. I said this to you the first night I came to you Shell: We spend our lives doing things we think will help us to achieve happiness. If I just had more money, if I just had the perfect partner, if I had a better job, I'd be happy. But, that's backwards.

Happiness isn't hidden away behind all those things. It's built in! It's a gift we're all given, but most of us don't take care of it and then we forget where we put it! I gave up searching years ago, Shell. I was just fine tuning. Everything I've been telling you about; those were just the tools I used to tighten here, or to loosen there. And that's my gift to you,

Shelly. I'm bequeathing to you my toolbox: it's up to you to take out those tools and use them."

"I will Jake. I promise. Oh, one more! I have one more question!" I couldn't believe I'd almost forgotten. Jake did a drum roll on my wardrobe door and beat me to it.

"What's the deal with the song, right? I think it might have wrecked your head for all of eternity if you didn't ask me. The reason you've been hearing it a lot since I died is because it was the last thing I ever heard. It was the song playing in the car when the crash happened. The reason it seems to be everywhere you go is because I'm still with you. Does that make sense?"

"Yes. It's just kinda sad to think it was the last thing you heard."

"Not at all! It was the best last thing I could have heard! Shure, I love that song: What could possibly have been a better choice to see me out?"

I nodded. It made sense, I suppose, though it was still a little difficult to see it from Jake's point of view.

"We came here for a human experience and we are only born into the one body, with the one mind and the one soul. We were born alone and we die alone. Be busy and successful at the business of life, Shell. Be responsible for your own adventure. You can't take responsibility for anyone else's."

I held up my hand, and he paused.

"I thought you said to be altruistic?"

305

"Yes, I did. But helping others to live their lives is different from trying to change them and live through them or live their lives for them. Do you understand the difference? Fill yourself up first. When you start to overflow – when you have so much life and joy that it's pouring out of you – *that's* when you can share more than just gifts or charity. Think of everything you want to say or do, every moment of the day, and think of that moment, as being your last chance to say or do it. Every moment counts."

"I know. Jake?"

17"Yes?"

"Thank you."

"Our time is up, Shell."

"I know. I know it's selfish, and I know you have to go, but I don't want you to."

"I am always going to be with you, Shelly. You know that. But I could stay with you because I had a purpose, and I've fulfilled that purpose now. You will do well, and you will live a good life. You're only getting started. When you heard *Galileo* last night, you realised that you'd always have me there in those words and that melody...and not just there. I'm everywhere. I'm all around you. But you don't need me anymore. You have goals and a purpose. Remember: you can't hit a target you can't see. Now you have targets. They're everywhere all around you too. So...do just one thing for me. I just have one request."

"What can I possibly do for you?!" I asked.

"You didn't think I was going to give you all this and not look for something in return, did you?" Jake laughed. I couldn't help it; I laughed too.

"Eh, well, yeah. I thought that was your job now!"

"Shelly, I'm going to ask you to do the same thing The Squire asked me to do: I want you to pass it on. All of it. Everything you've learned. I want you to share with others like I have with you. There's no point in having nice stuff unless you share it. And, remember, *always* remember: I love you."

And then...silence. Jake was gone. I woke up, and it was six o'clock on Monday morning. I sat there, in darkness and silence, but just for a few minutes. Slipping back into grief would have been an insult to everything Jake had given me. I got up, dressed and left the house, then took a slight detour on the way to The Gym.

I parked outside the graveyard. I walked to where Jake's body had been buried only a few weeks previously. I sat on the marble bench at the end of the grave.

"I love you too," I said.

*The End*